TAKE ONE ANECDOTE TWICE DAILY

TAKE ONE ANECDOTE TWICE DAILY

Dr Isidore W. Crown

The Book Guild Ltd.
Sussex, England

The Book Guild Ltd.
25 High Street,
Lewes, Sussex

First published 1993
Reprinted 1994

Set in Baskerville
Typesetting by Southern Reproductions (Sussex)
Crowborough, Sussex
Printed in Great Britain by
Antony Rowe Ltd.
Chippenham, Wiltshire.

A catalogue record for this book is
available from the British Library

ISBN 0 86332 882 2

CONTENTS

1

The Beginning

On a bitterly cold, rainy day, in January 1953, on the 12th to be exact, I started to practise in Peckham. To this day we remain in the same premises. Alterations have certainly taken place, as all the living accommodation has been taken over for practice use. Many years ago, the dining-room changed its use from eating to pen-pushing and became the practice manager's room; the bathroom became the practice nurses' room. The bedrooms became surgeries and a waiting-room. Alas, I could find no use for the coke-heated copper!

The garden, which was my pride and joy, now hosts two surgeries, a waiting-room, a receptionists' common room and a storage shed. A section of the garden still remains; the apple and pear trees refuse to be denied their share of the garden and still flower and bear fruit, as if nothing had changed.

All the stories in this book are true, they actually occurred exactly as I have described them, but to avoid embarrassment, where I have thought it necessary, I have altered the names of the patients.

Dear reader, should you recognize yourself even though your name has been changed, thank you for being my friend and making my life with you in Peckham such a happy one. I hope we will enjoy each other's company for many more years.

☆ ☆ ☆

I will open my account by actually mentioning one patient by name, Bill Godley. He saw me a couple of hours after I moved in, the electricity had not yet been connected and I saw him by candlelight. He has long since departed this life, but his family have evidently borne me no malice at the absence of light: his brother Fred and sister-in-law Charlotte are still with me after forty years!

For the first eleven years I worked single-handed, but to give myself a break from a twenty-four hour seven day week, from 1954, I employed the occasional locum. Indeed, I had already by 1955 built up enough goodwill amongst my patients to allow me to employ a regular locum for Saturday mornings; this enabled me to attend the sabbath services at the local synagogue. Besides giving me a rest from the workshop it also allowed me some time with my children. Patients who wished to see me personally on that day were able to do so at the evening surgery. I did a normal evening surgery.

One Saturday morning in February 1962, on returning home from the synagogue, this would have been about 12.30 p.m., I was asked by my wife to telephone the housekeeper at the surgery urgently: we were at that time already living in Brockley. We had moved from living over the surgery premises in 1958 as the living accommodation available had become too small for our growing family.

I telephoned the housekeeper and was astonished to learn that the waiting-room was crowded with patients, but the doctor had disappeared. Some of the patients had now been waiting for over three hours and she did not know what to do.

'Dr Watson didn't turn up then! He has never let me down before,' I remarked.

'He turned up all right, but didn't bother to do the surgery,' was the reply.

I could not believe I had heard correctly as the doctor had been paid for doing the surgery. I asked her to repeat what she had said, and she did. I then asked her to relate exactly what had transpired.

Dr Watson, who should have started my surgery at 9 a.m., had turned up late at 9.30 a.m., and appeared to be somewhat in a hurry. He had rushed into the consulting room to remove his overcoat, then walked into the crowded waiting-room and said, 'Hands up all those patients who are really ill.'

The astonished patients were mesmerised, and too shocked to answer. They just looked at him; no one said a word.

'Oh well, if no one is really ill,' he was reputed to have said, 'I don't see why I should waste my time.'

He walked back into the consulting room; put on his overcoat, said 'Good morning' to the patients in the waiting-room, and left. The patients were too bewildered to act; they did not know him and thought that he was playing a trick. It was not until they had become fed up waiting for his return that they had summoned the housekeeper. I was left tidying up the mess that day – with no lunch and no tea. I also did not get my money back from the locum.

By the year 1963, my practice had grown too large to manage single-handed and I took a partner, a very large, extremely pleasant Polish doctor – Dr Leslaw (Les) Kwasny. The practice, however, although increasing in patient numbers, did not grow fast enough to maintain two full-time doctors in style so after a couple of years together, Les decided to apply for a vacant practice in Dulwich. He wanted us to stay together, have the Dulwich practice as a branch surgery, but I thought the work entailed was too much for us to cope with.

We would have had three surgery premises: the practice he applied for had consulting rooms both in Woodwarde Road and Barry Road. This would have meant six consulting sessions a day – I still shudder at the thought. He decided it would be in his best interest to take the Dulwich practice and work it single-handed, so we parted. We still, however, remained the best of friends and often met and chatted, until his untimely death in December 1990.

I worked with locums and assistants for a short time after Les left while I sought a replacement partner, but finally gave up this chase, after an incident with a Persian doctor, in 1965.

Dr Mahan aged thirty, who bowled me over with his charm at the interview, agreed terms with me to accept an assistantship for six months – with a view to partnership. He really was every girl's dream of a young doctor: a charming fellow, tall, dark, handsome and debonair; a smile which lit up his face. He commenced work as an assistant four weeks before Christmas 1965. The patients loved him, there was only one way to describe his bedside manner – perfect. He charmed me, charmed my wife and, what was more important in my eyes, charmed the patients. He was a real asset, even in the short period of time before Christmas I already knew that he would make an ideal partner. Nothing was too much trouble for him.

Prior to his coming to work for me I had always been on duty on Christmas day, and he insisted, as he was not a Christian, he would prefer to be on duty for this holiday, and take the Persian New Year as a holiday instead. We therefore arranged that the morning surgery on the day after Boxing Day he would do on his own. This would allow me to return on that day from Liverpool; his being on duty would enable me to spend an extra day with my mother. Divine providence however told me not to leave an assistant on his own in charge of the practice, but to return with my family in the evening, on Boxing Day – in spite of the elements. It was snowing heavily when our car left Liverpool in the early evening and it continued to do so all the way to London. We arrived at four o'clock the following morning after a nine and a half hour journey – no M6 or M1 in those days – completely exhausted, but happy to be home.

At a quarter past ten that morning the telephone rang, an hysterical housekeeper was on the telephone. The waiting-room was full to overflowing and the assistant had not yet turned up. I rang him, there was no reply. I had however managed to snatch a few hours sleep so I dressed and rang the assistant again. Still no reply. It was fortuitous I had returned, it enabled me to go and do the surgery myself.

I tried several times a day for two weeks to get in touch with Dr Mahan by telephone, without success. It was always possible there was a fault on the line. I sent him a registered letter: the letter was never returned to me and I naturally assumed that he had received it, or been given it by someone who knew his whereabouts. I soldiered on alone single-handed for three months, when, out of the blue, I received a telephone call from this gentleman attempting to explain his absence from my surgery. He was most apologetic, still wanted the job, but had been in a hospital ever since I had last seen him, with ear problems. I did not bother to ask him whether he had been in hospital as a patient or a doctor, just asked him to come and see me.

He never did!

Some years afterwards, while reading a local paper, I saw his photograph. The chap was accused of having made amorous advances to a patient: he had a practice of his own. I followed the case out of curiosity and not surprisingly he was acquitted. He was such a handsome fellow, I would have taken a bet he was probably rejecting her advances, and she was seeking revenge.

After the Persian doctor fiasco I was left working single-handed once again, but as the workload was too heavy for one doctor, I decided to try to form a group practice. I was successful. Drs Bhatt, Blank, Cook and Healy agreed to join me in 1965, and for us all to practise together as a group, at 105 Bellenden Road.

Drs Cook and Healy intended to give up their premises in Hanover Park and Dr Blank decided to do the same in Choumert Road. Dr Bhatt however intended to retain his surgery in Bushey Hill Road; he was doubtful of being comfortable working with a group of doctors as he had always worked alone. Indeed, his decision was a wise one, he was uncomfortable from the first day; he left after a year, to return to his premises in Bushey Hill Road.

The group practice remains intact to this day although time has changed its members. Dr Helen O'Donovan joined us in 1973 and left in 1976 to join her husband in America. Dr Lai Cheng Wong, another lady doctor, joined us in 1983, Dr Anthony Stimmler in 1986 and Dr Michael A. K. Duggan in 1990. The only remaining partner of the original group is the author of this book.

Dr Cook's interest was psychiatry and as psychiatric patients do not behave normally we had problems in the surgery on dozens of occasions with his patients. Some of the experiences were frightening, many of his patients were psychotic; many had threatened suicide, some even went so far as to carry out their threats. Our good fortune was that no one actually carried out their threat on our premises.

One confused lady patient of his always came to the surgery to see him dressed in a different garb. I did not know the lady: on the first occasion I had the good fortune to see her enter the premises I was very respectful, I opened the front door to let the 'nun' pass through. On the second occasion I was in a state of shock: the same lady appeared a week later in the bizarre 'habit' of a fortune teller. I learned that her real profession was dipsomania, or could it have been pyromania, for she ended her life by setting fire to herself!

Another patient of his, an ex-nurse, always came to the surgery with a basketful of apple pies; she baked them specially for him. The surgery staff never refused her an appointment, always looked forward to her attendances for she was an excellent baker and Dr Cook always passed these pies around. They were very much enjoyed, until she decided her pies were much too good for this world and took them with her into the next.

Dr Cook loved to visit his weird patients, had a rapport with them; he spent hours chatting with what he called his 'nuts'.

One of his 'nuts', Albert, in his fifties, hated women; he only tolerated his mother and sister visiting him as they cared for his daily needs. He had not worked for years and had turned his flat into a 'pit'. When his family found it impossible to care properly for him, Albert's mother and sister turned to Dr Cook for help.

Albert had always treated Dr Cook as a friend, had always allowed him access to his flat without protest, so now this friendship was going to be put to the test.

Albert's family asked Dr Cook to arrange for Albert to be admitted to a psychiatric institution in whatever way he thought best. Whether it was to be as a voluntary patient, or compulsorily, was going to be for Dr Cook to decide. They just could not take it any more! Albert had decided to play his 78 gramophone records at full volume all day. They were deafened, so were the other occupants of the house, so were the neighbours. Albert had become a public nuisance and the neighbours had called the police.

Dr Cook went to see him, and as his friend, persuaded him that he should go into the Maudsley Hospital as a voluntary patient. After all the arrangements for his admission had been made, Albert suddenly asked Dr Cook whether, before going into hospital could he please phone the Queen and tell her what had taken place. This turn of events took the learned doctor by surprise, but he had no alternative except to agree. After all, Albert was going into hospital as a voluntary patient.

Albert disappeared into the next room to telephone the Queen, and was away, for what appeared to the anxious relatives to be hours: it was actually ten minutes. He then returned to inform Dr Cook that he had had great difficulty in getting through to her Majesty. Every obstacle had been put in his way by the palace staff to prevent her speaking to him. He was not to be put off, he had finally managed to speak to the Queen and asked her whether she wanted him to go into hospital. She told him there was no point in him going into hospital as there was nothing wrong with him, she did not want him to go, and as her loyal subject he had to remain at home.

Dr Cook had no answer – he did not want to end up in the Tower.

Dr Healy, who propped up the group alphabetically, always had the Irish charm, a handsome rugby player, who charmed all the ladies just by looking at them. In fact, although he is now in his seventies he still has this magic, a most even-tempered man with whom it has been my privilege to be associated.

Before he joined the group in 1961, I was waylaid by a patient of his in Highshore Road who complained to me that Dr Healy had not yet visited his mother. The fellow knew me because I was the doctor of other members of his family, and I was, at that particular time, going to visit one of them. He was furious, proceeded to tell me what steps he was going to take to make Dr Healy's life a misery; he even asked me for the address of the complaints' committee.

While speaking to the fellow, Dr Healy nonchalantly strolled up; I waited for the sparks to fly. He just put his arm round the man's shoulders and to my utter amazement, within three minutes, the man was begging forgiveness of Dr Healy for daring to call HIM to see his mother. The change in this man's attitude had to be seen to be believed. I now know why, when Dr Healy was so ill, so many prayers were offered by his patients for his speedy return and recovery.

Problems arose in the early days when I wanted to find some relief for half days or weekends. As there was no deputising service available I had to be on duty night and day myself. One evening in 1957 I arranged a meeting of some local doctors, to discuss the formation of a rota service.

The meeting was held in my home in Bellenden Road, and the doctors invited were Drs King-Brown, Knowles, Eppel, Cook and Healy. Drs King-Browne and Knowles practised in Asylum Road, Dr Eppel, who was the doctor of the Millwall football club, had a surgery in the Old Kent Road, and Drs Cook and Healy practised locally from a surgery in Hanover Park. This was the beginning of a night rota service for this practice which has continued ever since, although time has of necessity changed the membership.

I remember that night in 1957 when the rota came into being well. It was the first time I met Celestine Healy – Dr Healy's wife. She walked in, and Dr Healy was immediately the envy of every other doctor present. She looked gorgeous, had a perfect figure, and was an extrovert: she had certainly kissed the Blarney Stone. She was a magnet for every male because of her charms. Although a devout Catholic who went to mass every morning, for the Jewish festival of Tabernacles, Celestine cut fresh willow from her garden in Court Lane, Dulwich, to enable me to celebrate my festival; we became great friends.

She was a positive character; if she liked you, she loved you, and you became part of her family; if however she did not like you, she did not hesitate to let you know. Celestine was a genius in mockery, I have been in her company and watched people squirm in confusion as she turned her talents to their undoing. Poor Dr Healy often became embarrassed because of her forthrightness. One story of hers always amused me.

The husband of one of her friends had died, he was Jewish, but his wife, Celestine's friend, was a Catholic. The wife asked Celestine if she knew how she could get her husband's ashes scattered in a Jewish cemetery. I knew the chap who had died, he was a local GP, but I had never met his wife; in fact I did not know that he was Jewish until after his death. The fellow had made two wishes on his death-bed: one was that he was to be cremated, the other was to have his ashes scattered in a

Jewish cemetery.

Celestine knew that I was an Orthodox Jew and phoned me during surgery one day to ask me who to contact to fulfil the fellow's final wishes. I told her that I doubted whether this would be at all possible. Cremation I told her is frowned upon in Orthodox Jewish circles, and the Rabbinate would certainly not give permission to have his ashes scattered in one of the cemeteries over which they had jurisdiction. I was obviously not in a position to give her a definite decision, but told her to get in touch with the United Synagogue Burial Society.

She followed my advice and phoned the United Synagogue Burial Society. The secretary of the society, she told me, had been courteous and friendly, but told her that it was not possible for his ashes to be scattered in any of their cemeteries. She should get in touch with the Liberals. Her answer was curt.

'At a time like this, you have the audacity to bring politics into it!'

What the secretary had meant was that the Burial Society of the Liberal Synagogues do allow cremations and would have granted his wish. Unfortunately, the dying wish of the doctor had been specific: he wanted his ashes scattered in an orthodox cemetery. His ashes therefore still remain on a shelf in the crematorium office: awaiting the coming of the Messiah!

The last time I saw Celestine was on Christmas Day 1988, when I visited her in Dulwich Hospital. She had been a patient there for some time, and as I was on rota duty for the practice on that day decided to pop in to see her and comfort her. I knew that she would require it. She was such a religious person, missing her church on this special day would be a terrible blow to her morale. We always had a laugh together, and I was hoping my presence would help obviate some of her mental distress.

She was very ill, but I was not wrong; she still had not lost her sense of humour or sense of fun. My bleep went whilst I was at her bedside, and she burst out laughing.

'Progress has to take place,' she said. 'We never had anything like this in the old days. We could take our time then. Even our Christmases are machine spoilt. You had better get going!'

Sadly, she died a few days later.

2

Out of This World

It was 8.45 a.m. on an overcast, dark, dank, miserable January morning in 1987, the time when I normally set out from my flat in Forest Hill to drive to the surgery. It had been snowing for a couple of weeks and there was a foot of snow on the ground. Public transport had been disrupted, train services had been cancelled and the only means of travel in this part of London was the bus. Even buses went at a snail's pace, but at least they still operated. It really was difficult to get about, and people whose work was not essential were advised by the authorities to remain at home. Many did so, and found that their employers had other ideas: when they returned to work, found a day's pay had been docked for their absence.

I was unable to use my car to get to the surgery because of the thick snow, and decided to make the journey by bus. This meant a walk to the bus stop opposite Forest Hill Station, which is normally a ten minute stroll. Now, in the prevailing conditions, it would take me half an hour. Who cared? Everyone appeared so friendly; adversity seems to bring people together.

As I left my front door, I said, 'Good morning' to a girl who lived in the same block of flats; I had on many occasions raised my hat to her, but had never spoken. She was tiny, her little face showed through the mass of clothing with which she had protected herself against the elements. She smiled and attached herself to me for she too was walking to the station to catch a bus. I learned the girl was Japanese, and was studying English in Honor Oak Language School. She had no intention of letting me escape; she was obviously intent on practising her English on me for she kept up a continuous conversation as we trudged through the snow. Our main topic was Japan, and we spoke generally about the country and how the weather in Tokyo and London were not so dissimilar. She asked my profession: when she learned that I was a doctor and had a son in Singapore she asked why, when I was already in the Far East, I had never spent a holiday in her country. I explained that I had not yet been to Singapore, my mother who had settled in Israel in 1966 had only recently died, and I had spent all my vacations with her. I said that she would understand my position as the Japanese too paid great respect to their parents.

The girl stopped, horror struck. I was wearing a heavy overcoat, scarf, balaclava helmet, gloves and wellington boots. I also walked with a stick to make me aware of the need to pace myself, and walked slowly and deliberately. I must have looked an old man! She turned abruptly, looked me full in the face, and with her face only inches from mine blurted out, 'Your mother must have been very, very, very old!'

At that particular time I was convalescing from a recent heart operation, and as I hate the cold at the best of times probably looked as if I was in the eighties rather than the sixties.

My heart problem had taken me completely by surprise, I had never previously suffered any symptoms relating to this part of my anatomy. On the way to visit one of my partners in hospital, Andrew Healy, who was recovering from a heart operation himself, I had suddenly felt a constricting chest pain while walking across the road. Lynn, the practice manager, who had been accompanying me insisted on me having an electrocardiogram in Kings' College Hospital, before visiting our friend.

When we arrived at the hospital we found that Dr Healy could not be visited at that particular time as he was in the X-ray department. I therefore had no chance to prevaricate, just obey Lynn's instructions and have an electrocardiogram, followed by a little run on the treadmill myself. Andrew had not been expecting me. The look on his and his wife's faces seeing me wired up for the treadmill on Storks Ward when they came back was of complete and utter stupefaction. Storks Ward did have the dubious privilege in the following week of having both of us as patients at the same time. It must be some sort of a record, for two doctors, from the same practice, to be in the same ward recovering from heart operations at the same time.

To revert to my story of that January morning in 1987, I must have looked a sight to the patients in the surgery as I walked down the path from reception to my consulting rooms on that day. There were one or two patients in the waiting room as I walked through, and I remember passing the remark, 'Thank God it's warm in here!'

I went to my room, took off my outdoor clothes and wellington boots, and put on a pair of shoes. I was now ready for action, put a stethoscope round my neck, and prepared to commence my consultations. I opened the waiting-room door and beckoned to Alvin to come in. I had known him over thirty years, ever since he had arrived in this country from the West Indies. Alvin was a small balding West Indian man, who always came in to see me in his best Sunday suit. He treated me with the greatest respect even though I had told him on many occasions that he was a 'bloody nuisance'. He knew that in spite of my mannerisms I had a soft spot for him. In spite of his persistent backache he had still managed to work as a platelayer on the railway for over thirty years. Alvin looked at me as if I was not there. He did not move.

Exasperated, I said, 'Come on Alvin, you can come in now.'

He looked hesitant, dumbfounded, completely perplexed. He got up slowly from his chair and came into the room.

'What's up?' I asked.

'You're dead!' he stuttered. 'He told me you had a heart operation and died.'

'Who told you?' I asked.

'My friend Egbert,' he answered.

'What's wrong with being dead?' I asked.

I lowered my voice and whispered. 'Don't shout it out, but I died under the operation. They really messed it up. These hospitals are not the same as in the old days. They probably experimented on me knowing that I was a doctor and would never report them. They are a load of scoundrels. They know that they can get away with it. They are always trying new things on doctors, hoping they will work. You can't blame them completely, new treatment costs a lot of money so they give it to doctors first, but it doesn't always work. Anyway it was too late in my case, but the problem we now have is that you had a heart attack last night and you are dead too. It just has to be my luck to have to do casualty in heaven today, and you have to turn up. You always had a lot of problems when you were alive, I suppose you have brought them all up with you here. I never have any luck!'

He had, when he had come into my room, plonked himself down in the chair in a state of collapse. His face was ashen, not a muscle in his face moved. His body was limp, his eyes glazed, just stared into my face in utter disbelief. His lips trembled and moved uncontrollably, no words came out.

'Why did you come to casualty?' I asked.

He suddenly seemed to wake up as if from a trance, and his eyes wandered round the room. He was trying to recognize objects, but still did not say anything. He saw my old army photograph, which had been taken when I was in Crookham and which has been on the wall of my room for many years; this appeared to stimulate a reaction for he blurted out, 'You're joking!'

His brain and mouth however did not appear to coordinate; I could almost hear his brain ticking over saying, 'I recognize these objects, but I am not quite certain.'

The snow had started falling again, this gave the whole atmosphere an unearthly, eerie effect. The surgery is situated in a busy road, traffic is non-stop, background noise is continuous, now there reigned complete silence. The effect was funereal.

'You are up to your usual tricks,' he stammered, still in a kind of trance.

'Now look here,' I said, 'you are the one who said I was dead, you said so when you came in, I didn't volunteer the information.'

'I've got a terrible throat,' he said, in his usual expressionless manner.

This time he startled me. Whenever I had previously seen Alvin, and over the years this had been several hundred times, he had always been multisymptomatic. His head had knocked; his ears had buzzed; he had noises in his knees; in medical jargon he was psychosomatic, a hypochondriac, I had never ever seen his so quiet and uncomplaining, just to have one symptom. This behaviour of his was completely uncharacteristic.

I examined his chest, took his blood pressure, he still remained silent. His normal practice had been to speak all through the examination; I had always had to tell him to shut up whilst examining his chest. A regular consultation had usually ended up by my having to stand up and open the door to show him out; he took up so much of my time with the multiplicity of his symptoms.

Not on this occasion! He took a deep breath when asked to do so, and behaved like a model patient. I had never known him so quiet. I could tell from his reactions that I had not completely reassured him that we were both alive.

The stillness outside, no traffic in this normally busy area, certainly helped to add to his discomfiture. I could see he did not quite know what to believe. He had been so convinced by whoever had told him of my demise that my reappearance had been too much for him. I now felt it was my duty to reassure him. After all, I did not want to frighten him to death!

'I was only pulling your leg as I usually do,' I said, 'I was only joking, I am not really dead, I was only kidding.'

He stared at me for some seconds, he was trying to remember something.

'You don't have to pretend to me,' he said, 'You really are dead you know. I know that. Egbert told me. He went to your funeral.'

This was one occasion when I was stumped for an answer. I realized that whatever I now said would not alter the situation. Nevertheless, he was my patient, and it was my duty not to forget that. I had a duty to continue to reassure him.

'They must have buried the wrong chap,' I said, 'no one invited me to my funeral.'

He did not answer, took the prescription I gave him, stood up, opened the door into the waiting-room, and walked through it into the garden. He did not even stop to say goodbye.

I next heard a shout of pain and rushed outside. Alvin was limping down the garden path. He had kicked the garden wall to prove that he could feel pain and that he was still alive. He must have been so desperate to prove his point that he had kicked it with more force than he had intended. I watched him as he limped, moaning and groaning to the reception area. He had certainly done some damage. He came back to the surgery next day, not to see me, but to see one of my partners about his foot.

He still comes to the surgery, but I personally have not had another occasion to examine him. He avoids me like the plague.

He does not like ghosts.

☆ ☆ ☆

Jimmy, a friendly black man from Sierre Leone with a face wrinkled like a pomegranate, a grin which extended from ear to ear and never left it, lived in Crofton Road in 1977.

He had worked for the British in Africa as a railwayman. When the British gave his country independence he continued under the new regime, then, when he retired in 1975 came to live in this country.

He had one wife, she was a patient of mine until the

couple divorced, when she moved out of the area. He also boasted of several concubines whom he had left behind in Africa. I use the word 'concubine' in the biblical sense: Jimmy called them wives, but the wife who had accompanied him to this country always refused to accept them as wives.

These wives (concubines) had produced children for Jimmy. To his credit he went back occasionally to see them, and provided them with money, which on a pension he could ill afford. Although I asked him on many occasions why he had ever come to this country after he retired – he always grumbled to me about our weather – he refused to tell me. My original guess was wives trouble, but after getting to know him better I wondered in the end if it had something to do with witchcraft.

In 1979 he developed heart failure which resulted in my having to make many visits to his home and I got to know him very well. We became friends. By the time he had heart trouble problems he had divorced his wife in this country. I can't remember who instituted proceedings, but when the event I am about to relate occurred he lived alone, with only friends to attend to his needs.

He lived upstairs on the first floor of a house which had been converted into flats. In his dining-room were placed obelisks (small stone pillars about eighteen inches high) on the floor. There were about a dozen of them round the wall; to me they looked like small grave stones, and they were placed round the room in some sort of peculiar pattern. Not being familiar with African culture, perhaps not willing to question his beliefs, I at first pretended not to notice these objects. On becoming friendlier I began to question him as to the reason of the objects on the floor.

He now gave me a thirty minute lecture on African

culture, the part which the witch doctor played, and the nature of his performance. I learned that tribal Africans hated and avoided hospitals. Where a person dies is regarded by them as a place of bad luck, and as many people unavoidably die in hospital, it is a place of ill omen, best avoided. This perhaps explains why witchcraft still cannot be eradicated in parts of Africa.

I now learned the reason for the obelisks. They were something to do with his part-time work: he practised witchcraft. Many of his friends came to him to make use of his services; they came to him to cast spells on their enemies, and he obliged them. I listened to him spellbound: it was the first time in my life I had met a real-life witch-doctor, even though the witch-doctor was masquerading in western clothes. I was fascinated and intrigued that although Jimmy practised his beliefs, he still expected me to cure him. It was an eye-opener to me that Jimmy, whom I had always been given to believe by him to be a Christian, could actually believe in such pagan creeds.

I now asked him as a special favour to me, to cast a spell on my mother-in-law. She was someone I told him I could not bear the sight of. She was someone I would love to see suffer the same torments which she daily handed out to my long suffering father-in-law. If Jimmy were successful, I was certain when my father-in-law knew who his saviour was, he would reward Jimmy well. My father-in-law was a rich man, he would be much richer if his wife did not spend all his money. Jimmy had been wise to tell me his profession, I was about to make Jimmy a rich witch-doctor.

Jimmy listened to me without saying a word, then asked me my mother-in-law's first name.

'Sarah,' I said.

'How old is she?' he asked.

'About seventy, no exactly sixty-nine and four months.'

I had already got the message that witchcraft was a precise art and could not work on approximation.

'Dark or fair?' he continued.

'Dark.'

'Short or tall?'

'Short, about five foot nothing.'

'Round or oval face?'

'Round-faced.'

'Fine,' said Jimmy, 'I've got the picture, I will now put a spell on her for you. You've got to be exact in every detail, you know, you just can't put a spell on somebody unless it is the right person.'

Although we had become quite friendly, simply by the number of times we had seen each other, his understanding of English culture was evidently still not sufficient for him to understand my humour. He honestly believed I meant what I said.

He walked slowly to the cupboard in the dining-room and put on a funny sort of a white shirt. As he prepared to put on more regalia, I pretended to be somewhat apprehensive.

I said in a very loud voice, 'For God's sake, Jimmy, wait a second.' I put my hand on my brow as he turned to look at me, 'I forgot to tell you Jimmy, but my mother-in-law is a real old witch herself: is it possible that any spell you put on her might backfire?'

'What do you mean, backfire?' he said.

He was now putting on some funny multicoloured cloak; he had obviously not understood what the expression 'backfire' meant.

'I mean the spell you intend to cast on her will come back to you. I don't know enough about this witchcraft not to ask you this.'

He was struck dumb! I thought he would have a heart attack there and then. He went an ashen colour, ripped off the cloak he was putting on, took off the hat he was wearing, loosened his collar, became breathless and collapsed into a chair.

He refused to carry on. He remained seated. He was adamant. He would not put a curse on my mother-in-law in spite of all my pleadings. The belief in the supernatural is so great, even in the westernized African, that I had to spend a good deal of time afterwards in reassuring him. He also made me promise I would never in any circumstances mention his name or his existence to my mother-in-law.

I visited Jimmy many times after this episode, but never once did I ever allude to it; neither did he. He went to the grave in 1981 still believing that I was related to a witch!

Jimmy was not the only patient of mine who believed in witchcraft. I had a Nigerian patient in 1974 who told me that she would die in childbirth. The power of the belief in magic and voodoo is such that she had no doubt whatsoever.

A spell had been cast on her back home, and she was convinced no power on earth could now save her. She had been told by a witch-doctor in Nigeria that she would die in childbirth when her seventh child was born; this pregnancy was her seventh. I did not have the experience of Jimmy in 1974, and regarded her whole story as stuff and nonsense. How could any sane person living in England in the twentieth century believe such rubbish?

I performed all the routine ante-natal examinations right through her pregnancy, poo-poohed all her fears of dying, and sent her into hospital when labour commenced.

She had shown no symptoms of any abnormality

during pregnancy and I had no qualms in dismissing her fears. Besides, I had taken the precaution of giving her anti-witch-doctor medicine. This, to the uninformed reader, consists of mist. gent. alk. with twenty drops of acetophenatidine added, I have tasted it – it tastes awful. It made me vomit, but it works – I have never been plagued by any witches! No self-respecting witch could possibly come within a mile of anyone drinking this mixture. I was hoping that my pretence in prescribing medicine to combat her fears might have met with some success. I was wrong.

To my horror the midwifery sister of Dulwich Hospital telephoned me after having delivered this lady and said that my patient had been delivered of a normal baby, then died.

She had suffered a cardiac arrest after the delivery, with no prior symptoms. The baby had been born naturally, there had been no complications at the birth, and the second stage of labour had only lasted one hour. When waiting for the placenta to be delivered, the lady who appeared to be normal, had asked to see the baby. She had been shown a healthy boy, given the baby to hold in her arms, nursed it for a few minutes then collapsed. The midwife thought her attack was a simple faint, but it was not, her heart had just stopped beating!

They were unable to resuscitate her. Did I have any suggestions to offer? I did not like to be facetious and say that they should put the cause of death on the certificate as 'voodoo'.

I hesitated for a few seconds before I remarked, 'The only answer I can offer is voodoo.'

I expected a peal of laughter to follow my remark, but to my astonishment this did not happen. The maternity sister did not appear to be at all surprised at what I believed to be a statement of the utmost stupidity. She then told me that she had heard of several similar cases to mine, of patients who claimed to have been bewitched and died.

3

My Jamaican Pals

I had succeeded in building up for myself quite an established practice by 1963, and as many immigrants from the West Indies established themselves in the area a good number became patients of mine. I made many friends in the coloured community. I liked their Victorian values, their happy dispositions and sense of fun. I was not therefore surprised when Irving, a young Jamaican lad aged nineteen years, came in to see me in 1964 as an emergency.

He had only been in the country a few months, and had come to join his parents who were living in Peckham. They had been patients of mine since 1956, but he had remained in Jamaica cared for by his grandmother. This was not unusual at that time, I knew of many patients who had children cared for by their folks back home. The parents waited until they had made good here and established themselves before they brought their offspring over and in the meantime, Granny back home cared for the kids.

Irving's emergency was, he had an urethral discharge. His actual wording however was, 'It jooks me in my thingy!'

The terminology was explicit. I knew immediately

what he meant. I had by 1964 learned a good deal of the Jamaican expressions and his statement needed no further clarification. I examined him, but when I told him he had a venereal infection and that I would have to send him to a venereal diseases clinic, he became furious. I explained to him that I was sending him so that he could be investigated and treated properly, but my efforts to pacify him failed. He just became angrier and angrier. Finally I asked him to tell me his story; why my sending him for proper treatment was causing him such distress. I hoped that by telling me he would calm down.

He told me he had been solicited by a white girl at the corner of Rye Lane and Peckham High Street, outside Jones and Higgins, two nights previously. She had taken him to Peckham Rye Park, charged him ten pounds for sex on the grass and only allowed him to perform once. Now I knew as well as he did that ten pounds was a lot of money, and I could understand his distress at being told he had an infection. He had paid her his good hard earned money! She was white, how could she have possibly given him an infection?

His understanding was, having paid a white girl for sex, he would be free from infection. He had never stopped having sex in the West Indies, he could not remember how many girls he had been with, but he had never caught anything! It did not take me long to realize from the way he was describing events, and his discomfiture, I was dealing with a real 'thicko'.

I put on my most serious expression, which was a real effort at the time, and explained to him that ten pounds was a lot of money for a white girl to charge for sex in a park. He had to be someone special! With tongue in cheek, I told him that never in a thousand years would I have been charged as much as this, for a quickie in

Peckham Rye Park. It was just not on! He had definitely not been overcharged; this girl had fancied him. It was obvious: besides having sex with him, she had given him a present. In this case it was gonorrhoea. He was a very lucky boy.

If she had gone overboard, found him irresistible, she would in all probability have charged him twenty pounds. He would then most certainly have been given syphilis as a present. If she had charged him more than twenty pounds, God only knows what devilish present she would then have presented him with.

He was a very lucky boy to have escaped with such a small present, and the lesson he had been taught was that if he had to pay for it, he should do without.

While I was making my explanations, doing my best to keep a straight face, he stood looking at me open-mouthed, as though I was reading a tract from the Bible. How I thanked my grandfather and rabbinical teachers for giving me a grounding in the Talmud, and allowing me to argue a case without knowing what I was talking about.

Irving, I could see, was trying with all his might to absorb what I was saying to him, but was fighting a losing battle. I don't think he understood my reasoning at all, in fact I am sure he did not. He was not the only one, I did not understand it myself. His face had the same bland expression when I had completed my recital as when I had commenced, he was however suitably impressed. I had done my job.

He went away quite happily to St Giles' Hospital with my letter to the special clinic there.

George came in to see me for the 'thousandth' time, one

evening in 1975, complaining of grating in his head. From 1969 he had driven me to distraction with this grating; no treatment of mine had been of any avail. He had now come back to see me, for the treatment advised by the hospital I had last referred him to had been useless. I had already sent him to six hospitals and he was now referring to the seventh! In an effort to get him off my back, I had referred him over the years to various hospitals hoping that some bright consultant might accidentally hit on a cure – no joy.

I stared at him for a few moments, looked around the room, then got up and left, with an excuse that I had to see the practice manager on an urgent matter. I wanted to think, away from my torturer. I was now at my wits end! My diagnosis was, still is, that his symptoms were due to Eustachian tube catarrh, and as every doctor knows treatment for this condition is difficult.

George was a small, black, West Indian gentleman, aged forty-nine years who to his credit had, in spite of his symptoms, taken very little time off work. He was however a constant complainer, a thorn in my side, a weekly attender at the surgery, and I was never too pleased to see him, for I had up to now never given satisfaction.

I returned after having had a little breather and opened one of the drawers of my desk to take out a book which lists all the hospitals in the London area. This had been presented to me by the emergency bed service. I intended to send him to the furthest hospital in the book with some cock and bull story that it was the only one left which specialized in the disease from which he was suffering.

In the drawer my eyes fell on a screwdriver which I had evidently used for some purpose in the surgery and forgotten to take home. I knew that he was not too bright intellectually so I took the screwdriver out of the drawer, put it on my desk and waited for the reaction. There was none. The screwdriver was a large one, and for the life of me I still cannot remember the reason for it being there.

I took hold of George's head between my hands, and shook it sharply several times backwards and forwards. He offered no resistance, just allowed me to do it. I kept my hands on his head, then shook it smartly side to side.

'I've got it! I can hear it!' I said.

I pretended to look pleased. He didn't answer, just stared at me. I looked him straight in the eyes.

'I know your trouble, they have all missed it! The screw in the deep fascia connecting your parietal and temporal bones has worked loose. Why didn't you tell me that beside the grating you had a click?'

He just sat there mutely, not comprehending my argument. He was obviously more lost for words than I was, so I repeated the process. Taking his head between my hands, I shook it several more times, backwards and forwards, and side to side. He just sat in his chair bolt upright, allowing me to proceed, not uttering a single word.

The screwdriver looked at me so longingly that I took it, and pressing it gently into the area of the temporo-mandibular joint (jaw), turned it a few times. I made sure I was turning it correctly, clockwise, as one would tighten a screw, so as to avoid any suspicion. He did not flinch or show any emotion, so blinding him with science, I explained what I was doing to him. I was tightening the screw which fitted into a nut inside his skull, which had worked loose. To make sure he got the correct message I now put a little more pressure on the screwdriver, to cause a little pain. He got the message! He winced ever so slightly.

I then took his head in my hands and shook it again.

'Not quite tight enough,' I said.

I turned it a few more times, until he winced again. I stopped, then I shook his head again.

'That's better,' I said, and instructed him to come back every three months to have the screw tightened.

He had hardly moved during the whole operation except to wince, when I had put some extra pressure on the screwdriver. He had never been the brightest of persons, conversation had always been difficult, so his lack of conversation at that particular time was not unusual. The only topic we had ever discussed had been his grating; now that I had 'cured' it, he was lost for words.

I explained to him that he was one of those rare people who required this operation, and he would almost certainly never meet anybody with the same problem. In all my experience I had never previously met a case. He was lucky I read the *New Jersey Journal of Medicine* for a specialist in Memphis had written about a case similar to his. He was a very lucky chap he had come to me now; the specialists in this country had probably never come across a case like his.

I looked at him anxiously, waiting for him to say that my treatment hadn't worked, that I was a fake, but he just sat there uncomplaining, glued to his seat, staring at me. He then 'tried' his head.

'You've cured it,' he said. 'I've always told my friends you're good.'

With those few remarks he left me, only to return regularly every three months for five long years to have the screw tightened. Whenever I cleaned out my desk after our first success I made sure that the screwdriver remained in the drawer. I bought another one for home use.

On his last visit to me in 1980, he told me that he was leaving London and going to live in Birmingham, what should he do about the treatment? I told him to be explicit with instructions to his new doctor, the doctor would understand. He should tell his new doctor that he had a screw loose in his head in the parietal area.

I now only hope his present doctor has a steady hand after hearing my diagnosis. I also hope he has the right screwdriver to fit 'the loose screw'!

☆ ☆ ☆

The Taylors, a large Jamaican family registered with me as National Health patients in 1954. They were not really a family in the true sense of the word; they were a group of men who arrived in this country in 1952, recruited for jobs which we British were not prepared to do. These jobs, so called menial ones, were for bus conductors, hospital porters and dustmen. Being young, they were sexually active, the men not having their women with them found partners in Hyde Park who had sex with them behind a tree – for the princely sum of one pound.

As the young men became more prosperous they deserted Hyde Park and were catered for sexually in their lodgings by a pretty Irish girl who was looked after by a white English pimp. The situation was an interesting one; while the girl was performing her services, the white Englishman would spend his time in their lodgings selling them his Rael-Brook shirts, on the never-never!

The fellow was really a door-to-door saleman of shirts and only ran his sex-selling as a sideline. The pimp took this girl with him to all West Indian houses where there was business to be done in selling shirts and collars and at the same time earned himself an extra pound, tax free, from every customer who wished to be serviced sexually. The girl was only available to shirt-buying customers: no purchase, no girl.

The shirts he sold, Rael-Brook, were only available from him on hire purchase so he was sure of a regular clientèle, and the girl was just a bonus which gave him a tax free income. If you were a customer, you told the fellow when he called you wanted the girl's services, you paid him a pound, and you took the girl to your room.

Rooms were usually shared, landlords were difficult to find, and the rent of a room to a black man was always exorbitant. Most white landlords would not accept black tenants so black landlords had a field day and charged what they liked.

If your room-mate was in, he left the room for the few minutes you wanted to perform. The girl just lay on the bed, lifted up her skirt and pulled her knickers down. You had sex with her, the whole act only took about five minutes: she would dress and be back with her pimp as if nothing had happened within ten minutes.

Her pimp never left without an extra fiver in his pocket. How many houses he served in the same fashion they never found out. He would never leave without the girl. However hard these young men tried to find out where he lived, and on several occasions they traced his movements for miles, no one discovered his office or hideout.

An interesting incident relating to this family occurred in 1960 when they were drinking in a public house in Brixton. The family had by this time increased in number to include five brothers and several cousins who used to meet regularly once a week on Sunday morning in this pub. One cousin, Boysie, was white; an argument developed one Sunday morning amongst the family as to whose turn it was to buy the next round of drinks. The argument was a good-natured one, with much bantering, with the normal Jamaican sense of fun and humour, but which must have sounded offensive to people unaccustomed to the culture. Several black Africans happened to be standing at the bar that day, evidently listening in to the argument, unaware of the family relationship.

In their opinion, Boysie was being much too argumentative, authoritarian and condescending to his black friends. He was speaking to the black men as they understood a white American from the South spoke to his slaves. They were not prepared to allow their fellow coloured men to be treated and spoken to in this fashion.

Boysie, a thin faced, blond-haired albino, a scrawny chap, was the only fellow of the Taylor clan whom the Almighty had forgotten to provide with muscles. He must have weighed eight stone nothing, so it did not take much effort on the Africans' part to lift him out of his chair and hurl him out of the pub into the street.

The incident had happened too quickly and surprisingly for his family to prevent, but retaliation was swift and purposeful. Before the Africans had returned to the bar they were manhandled out of the public house accompanied by kicks and punches from the Taylor family. They fled, not knowing that black men can sometimes have white brothers. It is only a matter of how much melanin pigment is present in the skin.

I sincerely hope that they are wiser men now.

It was half past four in the afternoon on an unusually mild day in January 1970, when Sidney, a young six foot two inch Jamaican lad whom I had treated on many occasions previously, suddenly went berserk and smashed his way into the surgery. 'Smashed' is the operative word; he could not be bothered to turn handles, just used his brute force to get to see me. He flung open the front door – surgery consultations had already commenced – and on finding the door between the waiting-room and reception closed, smashed his way through it. This door was half-glazed, so the noise of shattering glass muffled a lot of his shouting as he propelled himself into the receptionists' room.

I left my room to see what all the commotion was about, to be confronted by an excited Sidney towering above me, demanding my presence to accompany him to have tea with the Queen at Buckingham Palace. His violent behaviour was quite uncharacteristic; he had always been a gentle giant and his manners had been impeccable. He worked in a printing firm and had also been doing a secretarial course at evening classes, but at that particular moment these facts were not the most important things to occupy my thoughts.

I looked at him in astonishment as he shouted to me over and over again that I should accompany him to Buckingham Palace. I realized that he had become acutely mentally disturbed: no one in Peckham goes to tea with the Queen without a written invitation!

Surgery had commenced, patients were already in the waiting-room, but if one is only five foot six and a half inches tall, not in the best physical condition, one does not if one is sensible argue with a chap who is over six feet tall, younger, more muscular, and in appearance very much fitter. I was also not in the best position to resist; he had me in a headlock, and was dragging me to the front door.

I now tried to humour him, but as he was asking for my company at the top of his voice, in the commotion I had no alternative but to shout back at him. He would not have heard me otherwise. He kept insisting that a taxi be called to take us to Buckingham Palace, but I reasoned with him – as best as I was able to do in the circumstances – that it would be quicker if we went in my car. After all, I shouted, we did not want to keep the Queen waiting!

I was told afterwards that the patients who had already arrived for evening surgery and were sitting in the waiting-room had decided that their ailments could wait for a more propitious occasion, and had made a very quiet exit through the front door.

When we opened the front door he saw my car and almost deafened me by shouting that I was right; we should go in my car, not wait for a taxi and be disrespectful to her Majesty. We got into the car. I had already made up my mind that I was not going to take any chances, that I was going to drive as requested. I must admit however it was distracting to have my fellow passenger singing 'God Save the Queen' over and over again at the top of his voice, deafening me. When we were forced to stop at a red light he thankfully did not ask me to ignore it; he just gathered strength and sang louder. Drivers of cars who had the misfortune of being at the side of mine at the lights gave us a quick look, and tactfully turned away. They obviously could not tell which one of us had decided to become so patriotic as to 'lose his marbles'.

I was terrified, wondered how the situation would resolve itself, but still had the presence of mind to drive along Walworth Road to the Elephant and Castle, then double back through the back streets of Camberwell, up Denmark Hill, to De Crespigny Park. He sang the whole time; by doing this I knew my driving through the back doubles had fooled him, and he had not doubted his belief in my sincerity that I was taking him to the Palace. The side entrance of the Institute of Psychiatry of the Maudsley Hospital is in this road and I was banking on the fact that he didn't know it. I was right!

I was hoping that when I had deposited him outside the Maudsley Hospital he would, believing that he was at the Palace, get out quickly, and so enable me to make a quick get-away. This was not to be. He insisted I get out first, and still tightly holding on to me, slid out over the driving seat. When we reached the pavement he changed his hold and grabbed me once again round the neck; not to hurt me, but to drag me along with him. It was a painful experience being dragged by a maniac, the force he was using for my compliance was excessive; I nursed a bruised neck for several days afterwards.

With his arm round my neck, shouting to bystanders that we were going to have tea with the Queen, we walked, rather he walked and I was pushed, into the side entrance of the Maudsley Hospital. The few bystanders who looked at us going into the Maudsley obviously thought to themselves those two are really going to the right place and kept well away.

I had only been to the Maudsley on one previous occasion; this was to take Mr Ward to the emergency clinic. This entrance was the main one in Denmark Hill opposite King's College Hospital; I was now lost. I did not know my way through the De Crespigny Park entrance, but I had now ceased to care.

There was a flight of stairs immediately in front of us, and since no one appeared to direct us to the Queen we, rather he, decided that she must be waiting for us upstairs. We went up the stairs, all the way up he kept singing 'God Save the Queen' at the top of his voice, and people in white coats kept coming out of side rooms telling us to be quiet. They came out, shouted 'Please be quiet', and disappeared before I had a chance to say a word. They made no effort to rescue me or to find the cause of the commotion. We had reached the third floor of this building when he turned and dragged me through some swing doors, and we found ourselves in a large waiting-room.

I still do not remember which psychiatric department we were in, except that we were in the Maudsley Hospital. I had chosen the hospital, he was now choosing the department and in my plight this was good enough for me.

The waiting-room was in urgent need of redecoration, not at all resembling a room at the Palace, but no matter, I told him, this was obviously not the Queen's room. There were chairs round the walls of the room, but they were all unoccupied. With his arm still round my neck, I told him that this was the booking-in room; guests had to wait here until the Queen sent for them. To prove my point I pointed to the other end of the room where sat a middle-aged lady receptionist behind a desk. She was taking no notice of us at all! She either must have been used to this type of behaviour, or was hoping that we were intending to make our presence felt in another department and were just passing through.

I now managed to persuade Sidney to lower his voice; we were obviously in a reception area in Buckingham Palace, and expected: the lady at the desk had taken no notice of us, she knew who we were. She was only waiting for the Queen to tell her when to grant us an audience!

In a hushed voice I now told him that it would not be right and proper for me to appear before the Queen without a wash. The drive in the car I told him had also disturbed my hair, I had to comb it to be presentable. I was in desperate need of a wash and brush up!

To my surprise he released me so that I could go to the toilet, and to my amazement he stretched himself full length on the floor, stopped singing 'God Save the Queen', and thundered out 'Land of Hope and Glory' instead. His voice was deep bass; this turn of events not only startled me but the receptionist too. She stood up, looked at me, then down at Sidney on the floor speechless and open-mouthed.

I didn't bother to explain my predicament to the receptionist or ask Sidney the reason for the change; I fled. It would have taken too long to explain the position to a hospital doctor had I remained; besides, I knew that I had a heavy evening's work ahead of me at the surgery. I had left my patient to be cared for in a most fitting place – the Institute of Psychiatry – a prestigious postgraduate psychiatric teaching hospital.

Instead of going to the toilet as he thought, I hurtled down the stairs to my car and fled to the surgery. I have never come down three flights of stone stairs so quickly in my life! Not surprisingly, I arrived back in the surgery in a state of extreme agitation, exhausted both mentally and physically, apprehensive at what Sidney's next move might be. His behaviour had been uncharacteristically bizarre; he was normally a docile creature and would never have put a headlock on me had he not flipped. He would in his confusional state probably not discover my absence for some time, but when he did, what would his reaction be? What would he then do? His mind had let him down, mine was in a whirl, I was terrified.

There was a waiting-room full of patients needing my attention when I arrived back, and I had no choice but to recommence doing or pretending to do a normal consulting surgery.

An hour later the inevitable happened. There was a telephone call from a doctor in the Maudsley Hospital informing me that there was a patient of mine, a man, causing a commotion in the reception area of the neurosurgical unit. The man was obviously abnormal, he was lying stretched out on the floor singing 'God Save the Queen' – Sidney had switched tunes again. This man when questioned, insisted that he was a patient of Dr Crown and was waiting for Dr Crown to reappear to accompany him to have tea with the Queen. The patient was adamant. Dr Crown had been with him when he came into the building and the receptionist corroborated his statement that he had entered her reception area accompanied by another chap. She could not be certain however who the other chap was, whether Sidney was telling the truth, or that the other fellow was indeed his doctor. At first he had the poor chap in a head-lock and afterwards, when he had let him go, she had only had a fleeting view of his face. The patient had only removed his headlock so that the fellow could go to the toilet, Sidney had told her so!

'Have tea with the Queen?' I pretended to be dumbfounded, 'I don't know what you are talking about. The chap must be mad! He needs to be admitted. If he is as barmy as that send him down to the emergency clinic and see what the registrar thinks about him. By the way, I would be grateful if you would let me know what you have done with him. If he really is a patient of mine I don't want to be called out in the middle of the night to a raving lunatic!'

This doctor with his clipped South African accent was a real nice guy. He rang back later to tell me that the chap in reception in the neurosurgical unit was a psychopath. When asked by the receptionist to stop singing and leave the premises, he had gone berserk. He had broken every chair in reception, smashed the desk, and attacked the nurses who had come to remove him. They had been forced to use a strait-jacket to restrain him, and the police had been called in. He had been admitted for treatment under 'police section'.

Sidney was in hospital for six months before being discharged, but I never had an occasion to treat him again. He had changed his address while still an hospital inmate, his family had moved to Deptford, and as his new address was outside my practice area they had changed his doctor.

Some years later when I was shopping in Rye Lane, this tall young Jamaican lad came up from behind and tapped me on the shoulder. I turned round, and there was Sidney beaming at me like a long lost friend. He had even recognized me from behind! He told me that his family had a doctor in Deptford as they now lived out of my practice area. I made no mention of our last meeting or whether he was having any treatment. He appeared to be completely normal, and we parted the best of friends.

My practice had increased in size so rapidly by 1961 that I decided to try out an appointment system and add a bit of prestige by employing a receptionist. For this purpose, as my first receptionist, I engaged Mrs Ellen O'Brien, a patient, an ex-nurse, who had been forced to give up nursing to cope with her two young children.

She worked for me part-time, but had previously been a staff nurse at King's College Hospital, trained in midwifery by Mrs Pretty, who was still at that time the sister tutor there. Mrs Pretty too was a patient of mine, and it always amused me when she came in to see me.

Mrs O'Brien just could not forget that she was no longer her pupil. She bowed and scraped before sister tutor, always addressing her as 'madam', but behind her back she called her 'Sister Pee'. At a much later date, when Mrs O'Brien had returned with her family to Ireland, Mrs Pretty herself became one of my receptionists and remained with me until she retired.

One of my Jamaican patients, Mrs Eubanks, who had arrived in this country in 1960, seemed to spend her life feuding with Mrs O'Brien. Mrs Eubanks called me out for visits to her children on the slightest pretext, and had a turn of phrase which always amused me. If one of her children was missing, not to be found easily, she would shout, 'Where you is?' When the child appeared, her raucous voice bellowed out, 'Where you was?'

I tried as hard as I could to get the lady to bring her children to the surgery, but it was a useless exercise. She just could not get used to an appointment system. The appointment system was in its infancy, and Mrs O'Brien had tried, without success, to make Mrs Eubanks understand that in order to see the doctor an appointment had to be made. Mrs Eubanks however cared nothing for appointments, or Mrs O'Brien; she had always managed to see me for her illnesses by gatecrashing.

The day arrived when Mrs Eubanks appeared at reception as usual without an appointment, but this time Mrs O'Brien had managed to give her an appointment for the same day on a cancellation. For some unknown reason the good lady did not attempt to gain immediate attendance; she kept her appointment. On leaving me however she frightened the life out of me, she told me, she had just had enough of that bitch at the desk, and was going to punch the 'filthy German bitch' in the mouth. She meant it too: she was a five foot nine inch, eighteen stone woman, and almost certainly packed a hefty punch. I pretended to be astonished.

'You don't know what you are talking about or you wouldn't say such things,' I said. 'Do you know who Mrs O'Brien is?'

I explained to her that it would be the most foolish thing in the world for her to attempt to punch my receptionist. Mrs O'Brien was not German as she believed, but Irish, and one of the leaders of the IRA in this country. It was obvious I told her, Mrs Eubanks knew nothing about the Irish, she would otherwise not have been so foolish as to even attempt to row with my receptionist. Should Mrs O'Brien be attacked she would have no hesitation at all in taking out the gun which she kept in her handbag and Mrs Eubanks would end up dead. Mrs Eubanks must have realized by now, I continued, that I myself was scared of my receptionist. My receptionist had been forced on me by the IRA. Mrs Eubanks should remember that I worked quite successfully without a receptionist before Mrs O'Brien came! What could a poor chap do when a gun was held at his head?

'If you still intend to punch her,' here I emphasized my remark by opening one of the drawers in my desk and taking out the book of death certificates, 'it will save us both a lot of time if I give you your certificate now.'

Mrs Eubanks turned an ashen colour, she had obviously heard about the IRA. What I had said, and the serious face which I had put on specially for the occasion, had frightened her. She turned and left me without saying another word; she wanted to get away from my surgery as quickly as possible.

I was curious to see what would happen when she actually came face to face with 'one of the leaders of the IRA' as she passed reception, I silently followed her. My curiosity was rewarded. As she came down the passage towards reception she went down on her knees, flattened out her bulky body, and crawled towards the front door like a woodlouse. She was going to make sure that she was below the level of the reception desk, out of view of the deadly Ellen, the 'crackshot' of the IRA.

Even though I had frightened her out of her wits she still remained one of my patients, but was now studiously polite to Mrs O'Brien. My concern had been that when she told me that she intended to flatten my poor receptionist she had a mental history for which she had at one time been treated in Jamaica.

It came as no surprise therefore when she cracked up again in 1967, became so disturbed, that I referred her to Dr Isaacs, the psychiatrist at St Giles's Hospital for treatment. I still however became involved in her treatment for I was called to the hospital one sunny afternoon to sort out a problem in which she was involved. She had been due to see Dr Isaacs on the previous day, but for some reason had missed her appointment. She had an inborn hatred of receptionists, and now proceeded to have a slanging match with the psychiatric receptionist at not being given an appointment for that same day, at a time convenient to Mrs Eubanks. The receptionist however had given as good as she got, had stood her ground, and given her an appointment for the following day. This was just not good enough for Mrs Eubanks.

Thwarted by the receptionist, she fled into the hospital grounds and began throwing stones at the ward windows. She had already broken a few windows, and no one sensibly was prepared to approach a tall, muscular, eighteen stone mad woman, armed with a handful of stones. The psychiatric department had determined by this time that there was only one way to deal with this menace – to have her sectioned and admitted to a mental hospital.

The mental act stated that two doctors were required to sign away her freedom. One doctor had to be her own general practitioner, a chap who knew her, would recognize that her behaviour was abnormal, and I had therefore been sent for on this lovely sunny day to sign the first part of the compulsory section order for her to be detained.

Fortunately, Mrs Eubanks and I had always had a rapport: when she saw me approaching she put her arm down, and stopped throwing for a second. She still had a handful of stones, and I was careful not to get too close at first. Mental people do behave abnormally! I shouted to her in the first instance from a distance, I did not want a stone thrown at me first. I told her that her stone-throwing was never going to get the required results. It was useless!

She waved me to come closer, and for ten minutes I became a stupid hero. I went up to her and explained that she obviously did not have the strength to break more windows, the ones that were left were now too high, and at too great a distance. If she would allow me to give her one of my muscle-strengthening injections she would be able to reach the top easily. She trusted me implicitly, gave me her bare left arm, and I gave her an injection of largactil – three times the normal dose.

It still took ten minutes of continuous talking before her responses became slower, and she became too drowsy to answer me. She then lay down, curled herself up into a ball, and began to snore. The two ambulance attendants almost ruptured themselves in lifting her on to a stretcher to remove her!

4

It Helps to be Jewish

I had not been in practice in Peckham very long before I realized how important Mr and Mrs Hood were to me both as patients and as friends. They lived in Maxted Road and were the apex of a pyramid of a very large family. Their importance as we quickly established a relationship was that they persuaded their family and many of their friends to become patients of mine.

Mr Hood, a man in his eighties, was a descendant of a long line of bookmakers, and seemed to know every racehorse, its birthday, its ancestors and how many races it had won. He knew every racecourse, every bend in the course and which horse would be most suited for a particular course. He had a library of books about racehorses, and whenever I visited he had one of these books open. These books fascinated me for they gave the ancestral tree of a horse, and reminded me of my school days, when I had to learn by heart the Kings and Queens of England.

His life had always been related to racing and his love of the sport continued until his dying day. I believe the only thing he did not know about horses from his books was the food they had at any one particular time. I could even be wrong with this supposition. Visiting Mr Hood one day my thoughts suddenly drifted back to 1951, when I had been an assistant in Newport, Monmouthshire.

I used to go to the synagogue every Saturday morning, and be accompanied part of the way home after the service by Sid Joseph, the local bookmaker. He had an office in the main part of the town and our walk took us through the castle grounds. The castle benches were always occupied by the 'local gentry', run-down types, who spent all their time looking through the racing papers picking out winners for the afternoon race meetings. Sid was a character, spoke Yiddish, and all the 'turf fraternity' sitting on the benches knew him and greeted him. For my benefit he would make facetious remarks to them and they would smile as he acknowledged them with a wave.

'*Du zest der mench*,' (you see that man) he would say, pointing to a tramp, '*ehr hut dus mihr gekaift*,' (he bought me this), and his hand would lovingly stroke the Rolex watch on his wrist.

One Saturday morning on our way home he suddenly turned to me and said, 'Put your shirt this week on Malka's Boy in the Wokingham Stakes.'

I had never heard of Malka's Boy or the Wokingham Stakes and was surprised that, knowing my feelings about horse racing, Sid had mentioned me putting on a bet. He went on, 'The horse can't lose you know, Isidore, my mother's name was Malka, and I am Malka's boy.'

'You know I don't bet, in any case I can't afford the money,' I said.

'Never worry, if it loses, it can't lose, it won't lose, but if it does, I promise you I will give you your money back,' he answered.

'I will ring you up after Sabbath to put my bet on,' I said.

'No you won't, I won't take your bet, ring up Shermans,' he said.

I did as he said on Monday, I put a pound each way on Malka's Boy which was running in the Wokingham Stakes that week. Sid was right! The horse won easily at 100-7.

On the following Sabbath when I mentioned my good fortune to Sid he just smiled and said, 'I told you so!'

Returning to Mr Hood, on his death bed, even though he was so dreadfully ill, he insisted I put some money on a horse which he was certain would win. He had broncho-pneumonia, was coughing up blood, but still had the sports page of his newspaper open with a list of the day's race meetings on his bed. Because he insisted, and to please him, I did something which I loathed, I got in touch with one of my patients, a bookie's runner, and put a pound on the horse.

One should always respect a person's deathbed wish. This horse did! It won handsomely at odds of 10-1. When I went back that evening to tell Mr Hood of my good fortune he just gave me a weak smile, with a certain look of disbelief as though I could ever have doubted his judgment.

He never gave me another tip: he died that night.

Mrs Hood, a frail little old lady was also in her eighties, and about eighteen months after Mr Hood's death she contracted influenza, which was followed by broncho-pneumonia. Treatment had not changed, and as she refused to be admitted to hospital I treated her at home as I had treated her husband, with twice daily penicillin injections. Unfortunately, her broncho-pneumonia occurred in September, in the middle of the Jewish holiday season.

I am an Orthodox Jew, and as Yom Kippur, a fast day, the most holy day in the Jewish calendar, was going to interfere with my daily visitation I was at a loss as to how I was going to cope with the situation. I had told Mrs Hood that I would arrange for another doctor to call, but she absolutely refused to hear of it. She would see no one but me.

We had built up a relationship of such trust even in the few years which I had known her that she refused to see my locum. We chatted it over and reached a compromise. I would give her an injection of long-acting penicillin immediately before the fast commenced, and I would give her another one on my return home from the synagogue, on the following evening. There was one proviso. She had to promise me that she was not to die under any circumstances. If she did, I would never forgive her, especially as I was going to pray for her recovery!

When I appeared after the fast, she looked in better shape than I did. I hadn't yet broken my fast. Her first words on greeting me were, 'You see I have done exactly as you asked – I didn't die!'

☆ ☆ ☆

Harry was old and ugly. He looked every bit of his seventy-two years. He had a scar the whole length of his face on the left side, and also sported an ugly looking deaf-aid.

I only saw him in the surgery on a couple of occasions for he was not really a patient of mine. He worked for a firm of bookmakers in the New Cross Road. As he did not live locally I agreed to see him when the occasion arose as a friendly gesture to his boss, Dave Moss, who was at that time the warden of the local synagogue.

I learned from Dave Moss that Harry was a bachelor. He lived alone and his whole life centred on going to

Bangkok on holiday – twice a year. Bangkok, in the late sixties and early seventies was not quite on the beaten track, certainly not in the cheap travel brochures. Only the truly wealthy could have afforded to take the trip: it would have needed a bachelor to save up his pay for half a year to be able to do so.

A few weeks after I first met him, he turned up in the South East London District Synagogue, New Cross Road, on the Day of Atonement. The Day of Atonement (Yom Kippur), the most holy day in the Jewish calendar, is a long day of prayer and fasting. The morning service commences at 8.30 am or thereabouts, and services continue non-stop throughout the day until sunset, when the fast ends. There is therefore ample time during the day for the not-so-prayer minded to hold conversations with their neighbours.

Harry, to his credit, remained all day. He could not read Hebrew well and must have found the services extremely tedious. During that first Yom Kippur afternoon in 1968 he made friends with my sons who were sitting next to him, and proceeded to show them photographs of Thailand.

I was sitting in the row immediately in front of them and my sons took it upon themselves to interrupt their father's prayers, to show me these photographs. They were enjoying themselves, having a break from praying, yet could not be accused of playing. Most of the photographs Harry had taken himself; included in the views were several of a beautiful Thai girl; he told them she was his girlfriend.

The girl looked in her twenties and the photographs included pictures of her children. They were most certainly not his! Their appearance was that of native Thais. Among the photographs were pictures of her parents and their village in the north of Thailand. He had not yet visited the parents in their village as it was a long way from Bangkok. He was saving up, and hoped to be able to do so on his next trip.

There was one photograph however which was missing, that of his girlfriend's husband. He was quite happy to admit that she had one and this did not appear to disturb him. He had no intention of marrying the girl, just befriending her. He had met his girlfriend in Bangkok in a bar, she had been working there as a hostess and the snide remarks of people when he told them this, did not seem to offend or embarrass him in any way.

I saw him again in the following year – he never attended synagogue except on Yom Kippur – and in that year the girl's family had grown; this had meant extra presents. He had now to include her sister and the sister's husband amongst the recipients of his beneficence, and arrangements had been made by his girlfriend for him to see them on his next visit to Bangkok. He then produced more photographs of Thailand including the parents' village where he had spent a weekend. In the photographs the village looked gorgeous, but his description of his visit there gave a different slant to the pictures.

The parents lived in a hut on stilts, with no proper sanitation. Even he was forced to admit that he was glad to get back to his hotel after a weekend there. The hut stank, so did the village, and the food was diabolical. He had not been able to eat any of their cooked food and had lived on a diet of fresh fruit. The people however had been so friendly, their hospitality had even made the smells bearable.

He returned to the synagogue on the following year with yet more fascinating stories of his visit to Thailand. I really felt very sorry for him for he appeared to have no life at all in between these visits. He never mentioned any friends in London, and I never heard him speak of any family whether alive or dead. It would appear from his life-style, the only affection he had ever received in his whole life was from this girl. She and her family were obviously giving him love for the financial benefits they obtained from him. His belief in their sincerity was such that I would never have said anything to destroy it.

In the fourth year he never returned to the synagogue and I asked his boss where he was.

'Silly old fool went to Bangkok in June and dropped down dead on the dance floor!' he answered.

☆ ☆ ☆

I had been in practice in Peckham only four days when Mr Thompson came to consult me. He had been on the list of my predecessor, Dr Morgan, and although he had been receiving treatment from the locum practice since Dr Morgan's retirement, he had decided to try a new friendlier face.

Mr Thompson was an ailing man in his middle fifties, who suffered from rheumatoid arthritis, asthma, chronic bronchitis and emphysema. He was therefore a frequent and regular attender at the surgery. I can even remember the first prescription which I gave him: it was for a new pump, and Rybarvin solution to put in it, to relieve his wheezing.

He was married, with two teenage children, and when he first came to see me, he and his family lived in Lyndhurst Way, round the corner from the surgery. When they moved to a house in Crystal Palace Road in 1956 he found the walk to the surgery just that little bit too far; he then came to the surgery in his van which he parked outside. In those days there were no yellow lines to prevent him from doing so. Few people had cars in the

50s and 60s, and there was always plenty of parking space when he came to see me.

I often wondered why he had a van not a car, but thought it impolite at the time to ask him; in any case it was none of my business. I thought he was borrowing his boss's van, but if so, could not understand why there were no markings or advertisements on its sides. No one who saw this van could have had any idea what the van was being used for.

One day, on returning from a visit just before commencing evening surgery, I found the van parked outside my door. I was not too pleased; he had expropriated my parking space. There was a noticeable smell coming from inside the van, and as I stopped and wondered where I had previously encountered this odour, it struck me. I had helped my *zada* (grandfather) in the *schechthouse* (slaughter house for chickens) as a young boy. I have never forgotten that smell.

My *zada,* a man in his eighties, had been a *shochet* (ritual slaughterer), and I had accompanied him on numerous occasions and watched while he worked. He had been most particular not to cause any suffering to a bird; not only had he been an extremely religious man, he had been a professional one too. The duty of a *shochet* is to slaughter an animal or bird without causing pain or distress: when on one occasion due to age, he was eighty-two years old at the time, he thought his hand trembled a little, he might have caused suffering, he retired on the spot.

The smell in the chicken house was the same smell as emanated from the van, but rather than embarrass Mr Thompson, I refrained from mentioning the stench. I did not have the heart to tell him that his van had a fowl, foul smell.

Mr Thompson continued to see me regularly in the

surgery until 1969, when he had an attack of influenza and was forced to take to his bed. As he was a chronic bronchitic the influenza floored him, he was so very ill that I was asked to visit him at home.

During the whole of the time I was in the house the telephone in the living-room never stopped ringing. It was answered by his wife, who appeared to be writing down orders, and was using the living-room as an office. I prescribed for my patient, told him that he would have to remain in bed for a few days, that I would revisit, but forbade him to make any attempt to go to work.

Whilst giving him instructions, I could hear his wife saying on the phone, 'Yes Mrs Cohen, No Mrs Cohen.'

I was intrigued: I asked him what his business was, and pretended this would have some bearing on the length of time that he would be housebound. He looked at me for a few minutes without answering, then, as I stood by his bed not making any effort to leave, he told me his story.

He was a poultry man, who bought his chickens from a farm in Kent, and delivered them to his clients in his van. He only dealt in dead birds, not live ones. When specially ordered, he delivered eggs as well.

'If you are doing a delivery service, why don't you advertise?' I asked.

He laughed, 'If I advertised, I would be bankrupt in a week!'

I looked at him in disbelief. 'Why?' I asked.

'I will tell you, if I can swear you to secrecy,' he answered.

I promised. He told me. His business was delivering poultry and eggs to Jewish clients in North West London. These clients were wealthy, always having parties, and his business was a flourishing one. Most of his clients however pretended to be observant, to lead good *kosher* lives, and 'You have now guessed why I have no markings on my van. My poultry is not *kosher*,' he said.

His business had to be run strictly by telephone and recommendation. He always delivered his poultry at the back door, never the front. Always to the lady herself, never to the maid or *au pair.* If the maid answered the door, he asked for the lady of the house. If she was not in, he gave the maid a dozen eggs, told her her mistress had ordered them, and that he would call back later to see the lady for payment. This gave him the excuse he needed to call back and deliver the poultry. He could not leave the poultry with the maid; she was never a party to the act. Indeed, the maid was always a worry to him and should one ever become suspicious, his business could be in ruins. At that moment, I thought a funny look crossed his face, but on reflection, it must have been pain from his wheezy old chest. He knew his role by heart. One mistake would cost him his living. As his clients trusted him implicitly, he would never betray that trust. He himself was not breaking any laws, he told me, he was only making a living.

His instructions were explicit. Should any rabbi or synagogue official be in the neighbourhood when he called, he was to postpone his delivery until the coast was clear. He had done his homework, made it his duty to recognize the *kosher* butchers in the area, also the local rabbis and synagogue officials. His deliveries were always made very early in the morning, or when it was dark. He therefore preferred the winter, he had longer periods for 'safe delivery'.

He quipped, 'I have often delivered my order by the back door, and as I have left, have seen the *kosher* butcher pull up at the front.'

'Why should the people bother to go to all the trouble

to buy from you?' I asked.

'Well,' he answered, 'if you are not too fussy yourself and want to pretend that you only eat *kosher*, you order meat and fowls from the *kosher* butcher weekly, but get your main supply of fowls from me. Don't forget my stuff is a quarter of the price of your *kosher* stuff. My customers save pounds by buying from me. My instructions are clear. Never ever provide a bill, give a receipt, or receive cheques. Telephone calls and cash only. My whole business depends on complete and utter secrecy. As I have already said, I would go bankrupt if I advertised, or anyone found out what my business was. If anyone ever became slightly suspicious and tried to trace my van, what chance would they have of following me, from North West London to Peckham?'

Mr Thompson had obviously been most reluctant to tell me this story previously, he knew that plucking feathers was not helpful for his asthma, and he also knew that I was a religious Jew.

'If this is all true, tell me the name of the rabbi in Wembley,' I said.

He had previously stated that he knew all the Jewish officials in the area which he serviced.

He didn't hesitate, 'Rabbi Myer Berman.'

I was nonplussed. He even knew his first name. He was right. I knew the rabbi personally. His story was true!

In 1972, Mr Thompson made peace with the rabbis and synagogue officials of North West London. He had an attack of broncho-pneumonia from which he never recovered. He died, and his business died with him.

Being Jewish, I have always taken Christmas Day for duty rota so as to enable my colleagues to spend this time with their families. Many of my patients have reminisced to me at times of details of my visits to them on that day.

Mrs Boulter, whose son always appeared to have an attack of asthma caused by the excitement of Christmas, remembers one Christmas day twenty-nine years ago very well. Master Boulter had been given a present of a train set, and promptly had an asthma attack. I was called to treat him and played with him and his train set for so long she believed his symptoms improved more from the playmate than the medication.

I made it a rule in the 70s on Christmas Day, to visit Mrs Tolputh, an old lady in her eighties, who lived in Brayards Road. Her house on two floors, alongside the railway embankment, was in a very dilapidated condition. The ground floor consisted of a dark dining-room, the window of which was only ten feet away from the grassy slope on which ran the railway line, and a small kitchen the size of a postage stamp. A door led from the kitchen to the cold, small, miserable outside toilet. The upstairs accommodation consisted of one small living-room-cum-bedroom. This was furnished with a single bed, a table and two chairs and a large old-fashioned wardrobe in the corner. A small coal fireplace with a wood surround completed the furnishings.

Every time a train went by the windows rattled, the foundations shook, but the house heaved a sigh and returned to its base: it was built in the Victorian period when houses were built to last.

She lived alone; although her son and his family lived only ten doors away the only contact she had with them was when her son dropped a card in her letterbox on Christmas Day. Her son was married, had two sons himself, neglected her completely, and never gave her the pleasure of seeing her grandchildren. She had no photographs of them, would have had difficulty in recognizing them for the last time she had seen them they had been babies. The reason the old lady gave for their neglect was that her daughter-in-law didn't like her. Not even to invite her for Christmas was beyond my comprehension.

I always believed I gave her a little happiness; she was such a dear sweet soul I could not understand why her family could not show her a little charity. I never found out when the family rift had occurred or why, but as her son and his family were not patients of mine I had no opportunity of asking them. Poor Mum was so lonely on Christmas Day, the streets were deserted: even the house did not vibrate to the shaking of the trains to break the silence.

An hour or so of my time for a sherry and a chat on Christmas Day was certainly no hardship for me.

One year, in one of these chats, she said to me, 'Do you know I met my son out shopping in Rye Lane a couple of weeks ago. I haven't come face to face with him for seven years. He looked so old. That battleaxe of a wife has certainly aged him. He was evidently shocked to see me for he said, "Good God, Mum, they told me you were dead." '

I looked at her rather sadly, but she was not at all put out.

'I really told him!' she said. 'A fine son I've got, he couldn't even come to his mother's funeral!'

His father was a rabbi, but Daniel, although religious, worshipped speed. Daniel was a young eighteen year old tearaway, a heap of fun, but so fearless as to be positively dangerous both to himself and to others. He was adventurous to the extreme; when our cat was stranded at the top of a poplar tree at the bottom of our garden in Brockley in 1964, before sending for the fire brigade we sent for Daniel. He thought it great fun climbing the tree like a monkey, rescuing the animal. The only reward he received from the cat for saving its life was some scratch marks on the back of his hand; from me, an anti-tetanus injection.

He rode a bicycle, was very proud of the speed he could obtain from it, but it was never fast enough for him to be able to try to kill himself on it. In 1965, when he managed to get a wage rise at his work in the jewellery trade, he bought himself a motorbike. Now he really could travel!

Unfortunately, he had only been able to buy himself a 250 cc bike for his money had only stretched this far; with this he was not too happy. This bike was not fast enough. In 1966, he had another wage rise and gave his motorcycle in part-exchange for a 500 cc bike; it was still not fast enough for him. He waited for another pay rise then bought himself a 1,000 cc bike. Now he was happy! This was the bike of his dreams!

What better place to test his bike than Pepys Road, which starts at Avignon Road in Brockley, and dips down in a steep hill all the way to New Cross.

The story of one fateful journey of his in 1966 I will never forget. He had actually come to my home to chat up our *au pair* but, finding her busy, had been forced to content himself with my company for some time.

'I was coming down the hill in Pepys Road, not too fast, earlier on,' he said, 'when I saw on the other side of the road this old geezer coming up the hill in a Morris Minor. I thought what a smashing way to test the bike. I turned on the throttle, the bike roared smashing like, just like an aeroplane engine. I crossed quickly to the other side of the road, raised the front wheel of the bike, went over the bonnet of the old geezer's car, over the roof, down on to the road without a scratch. You should have seen the face of the old bloke as I went over his head: I thought his eyes would pop out!'

By the way, this feat was performed by a lad wearing just a sports shirt and trousers without a helmet – protection was not compulsory at that time.

I however only half-believed his story: although I knew he was capable of doing almost anything I could not really believe that he had actually performed this stunt. He was known to exaggerate his exploits and I thought that this was one of his exaggerations.

You can imagine my astonishment on the following morning in the surgery, when this 'old geezer', a patient of the ripe old age of forty, came to see me with this remarkable story.

'You won't believe me!' he said. 'I was minding my own business, driving up Pepys Road from the New Cross Road early yesterday afternoon, when this mad lunatic came down the hill on a motorbike. He must have been doing over 100 miles an hour. This madman swerved across the road, climbed over my car bonnet, over the roof, down on the other side without falling off or turning a hair. He must be a raving lunatic, doc! People like him should be locked up!'

I insinuated he might be exaggerating, but all he said was that I was just like everybody else. No one believed him. Could he please have some tablets for his nerves? He was beginning to think he was imagining the whole episode, nothing had actually happened. I suggested to him that if his story were true, the motorbike must have damaged his car. His answer was a pointed – 'No!'

The bike was going so fast it had run over the car as if the car was the road itself. He had seen the same thing done at a circus by a stunt rider, but until yesterday had never believed it possible for this to be done on a normal road. He complained he had not been able to stop shaking since the incident, had not been able to sleep, and had not been able to work.

I certainly did not divulge that I knew who the culprit was, but asked him where his car was now parked.

'It's outside,' he said.

I now suggested to him that if we went outside to his car and looked for any damage we would almost certainly find a small scratch or indentation. The incident had only happened on the previous day and the motorcycle tyres must have been in contact with the car at some point. It was just not possible for a bike to have been airborne all of the time and it must have touched the car at some point to have been able to go over the top. We had to find something if he was telling the truth.

He looked crestfallen, but reluctantly agreed. We went on our tour of inspection, and when I pointed out to him a small scratch on the bonnet and a small dent in the roof, he became wild with excitement. Someone believed in him! The incident had actually happened! He was so relieved, he flung his arms round me and kissed me.

5

Army Tales

In 1950 Mike was a young single man when he served in Malaysia, or Malaya as it was then called. He was caught up there in the fight against the communists after the 1939-45 war. The only effective opposition during the Japanese occupation had mainly come from the Chinese communists, and they were in the field and armed when the Japanese surrendered. They continued their guerilla operations after the war ended, and Private Mike S..... was one of our many soldiers stationed in Malaya to keep them at bay and allow a legitimate government to consolidate its position. He was stationed in Jahore Baru near Singapore, and claims to have marched the length and breadth of Malaya during his army service.

He was a virgin soldier when he left the United Kingdom, and on leave one day decided that he had been virgin long enough. His friends had chided him unmercifully about his celibacy. Opportunity was plentiful in Malaya to remedy this, one day he was persuaded to visit the red light district in Kuala Lumpur after which his friends informed him he would return a wiser and more intelligent man.

He duly went to Kuala Lumpur, went to the red light district, and met a girl there. He was in uniform, and although the girls who worked the area knew it was out of bounds to the troops, what did they care? They were not going to be punished if found entertaining a soldier; besides, they always charged more for their 'services' to the services.

The girl who had picked him up, took him to her room on the ground floor of a run-down house, in the run-down area of Kuala Lumpur. He paid his fee, she drew the curtains, and he got undressed. He had been warned by his mates to protect himself from infection and he had taken the precaution of taking his own condom with him. Completely naked, raring to go, his penis as hard as a rock, and with his contraceptive sheath half on and half off, there was a knock on the door.

The girl was already lying on the bed waiting for him: at this point, as he was telling me this story, he could not contain himself and burst out laughing.

'What a situation to be in, doc, on your first time!' he said.

He was sweating like a pig at the time, but as the temperature in Kuala Lumpur was in the nineties he could not remember whether it was due to randiness or weather conditions.

The girl jumped up to see the reason for the knock and on opening the door shouted, 'Redcaps!'

Redcaps is the well-known name for the military police.

The girls who worked the district, the Redcaps, and the troops in the immediate area were not the only ones who knew that the red light district in Kuala Lumpur was out of bounds to British troops – Mike also knew.

He was not however without initiative. Completely naked, he grabbed his cap, trousers, shirt and boots, opened the window and jumped out. Being naked gave him a head start. He easily managed to 'out strip' the

Redcaps chasing him. Even today however, he bemoans the loss of his money.

'I lost my money, but not my virginity,' he moans.

He however can boast, 'I must be one of the few chaps chased by the Redcaps, completely naked, holding my cap, shirt, trousers and boots in one hand, and a sweaty French letter in the other.'

☆ ☆ ☆

Mr Norton moved to Camberwell Grove, a very prestigious road with many Nash houses in it in 1945, and he has lived in the same house ever since. I first met him in 1954. Mr Brean the local chemist whom I had known whilst working as a trainee assistant in Colindale in 1950 recommended him to me. Mr Norton's son Patrick at that time had glandular fever, and as he was dissatisfied with the treatment he was receiving, rather the lack of it, he transferred his family to my medical list. To be perfectly honest, there is still no treatment for glandular fever except rest and treatment of any secondary infection, but his previous doctor had been too dismissive of Patrick's high temperature and the Nortons' obvious concern.

Mr Norton was born in Brooklyn, New York in 1912, and admits to being a real tearaway as a young lad. He had run away to sea as a cabin boy when he was fourteen years old and as the ship docked in England, decided to stay here. His wanderlust however had not disappeared, and he moved on to Scotland where he managed to find a job. He settled down and persuaded his parents to come over to join him. They however did not like the life in the old country and went back to the States: as he refused to join them they left him here to live on his own. He managed to make a living by finding himself employment first as a moulder in an iron foundry, then a butcher, and finally as a labourer.

In 1938 he joined the International Brigade who were fighting in Spain; it was there he got his military experience which served him in good stead later on in his life when fighting for this country in France in 1940. He went to Spain because at that time he was very friendly with an Irishman from Tipperary. In his own words, 'we knocked about together', and it was a mutual decision to join the Spanish Republican Army. They stayed together until fighting in the Pyrenees in Spain they were separated, and he has never seen this man again. He believes his friend was killed in action; he made every effort to find him after his Spanish adventure without success. His sojourn in Spain in any event only lasted six months when he was forced to flee the victorious army of General Franco and return to England.

He could find no regular employment so volunteered for the British army. He now found that as he was not of British birth he was prevented from joining a regular service corps. As a foreign national he was allowed to serve in the Pioneer Corps; he joined the Pioneers where he served as a regimental policeman.

He was sent to France in October 1939 with no rifle, no ammunition, no military training, but with a set of toothbrushes. These toothbrushes proved to be invaluable when he was captured by the Germans in Boulogne in 1940.

The first time he handled a rifle in France was when the Germans attacked Boulogne on 10 May 1940 and a rifle was thrown into his hand. He was told to use it as best he could! His previous experience in Spain now came to his rescue, otherwise he would not have known how 'to load the blessed thing!'

His unit never had a ghost of a chance against the

German tanks and he was wounded and taken prisoner. He, and another 150 prisoners-of-war were then penned like cattle in Boulogne railway station for four days without food, before being force-marched through Belgium on their way to Germany and a prisoner-of-war camp. On occasions they were so hungry they would boil bullrushes collected from the roadside in a tin helmet to make soup. This strange macabre diet caused poisoning to so many of them that diarrhoea was the norm rather than the exception.

He had been wounded in action, this finally led to paralysis from the waist down for many months and being hospitalized. His condition at that time was considered serious enough for him to be admitted to a German hospital, and he was sent to Cologne. He was admitted to the hospital there under the care of German doctors and could not complain at the way he was treated for the three months that he was a patient there. Unfortunately, he did not improve, and as the Germans had no intention of continuing to use their scarce precious resources on a British prisoner-of-war, he was sent to Buckholt; this was more or less a holding camp.

One day, a doctor from Sweden whom he had previously met was passing through the hospital of the camp, and Private Norton complained of the treatment he was receiving. 'That goon there,' he said, pointing to a doctor, 'Called two orderlies to whip me out of bed and give me two crutches. He insisted they get me to walk. You know my case, you know I can't!'

The Swedish doctor reprimanded the German doctor and Private Norton, seeing that the moment was opportune said, 'Call this a hospital! There are no sheets, no pillows, just hessian mattresses filled with straw.'

That evening, every one got sheets and pillowcases.

From Buckholt he was transferred to a prisoner-of-war camp near the Dutch border. As he was still not able to walk, and still had to be carried everywhere by two other soldiers, he was transferred to Obermann prisoner-of-war camp. Here, for the first time, he was treated by English doctors.

The Red Cross now became involved, and he is the only person I know who was repatriated by them in October 1943 from Seela to Sweden. From Sweden he went on a Red Cross train to a hospital ship *The Empress of Russia* which sailed to Scotland.

A German seaplane accompanied their boat during the whole journey to Scotland and to this day he does not know the reason why. From Scotland, he was transferred to Sheffield Hospital for treatment, and he was finally discharged from the forces on medical grounds in January 1944.

While a prisoner-of-war he remembers being in fourteen different camps, but as we are writing of events which took place fifty years ago he has long forgotten their names.

His release from the army ended his longing for adventure and a new life opened up for him. He became conservative in his outlook and became a diamond polisher in Hatton Garden. He spent the next thirty years of his life there, until he retired.

Grandma and Grandad Hedge were well-known to my children: perhaps it was for their good nature, perhaps for their friendliness, but more likely for the provision of chocolate whenever they met.

Grandad Hedge when he retired in 1963 became my gardener, and the habit of giving chocolate now invaded my house; he never appeared at my home without a bar of chocolate for the children in his pocket. He loved children, had patience beyond measure, would sit on the steps in the garden and tell my two younger children, Simon aged six, and Shani aged three, stories of his exploits in the First World War. When my daughter became bored she would go to her swing, he would follow to push, and while pushing continue with his story telling. He would get carried away with his memories -he was probably only too pleased to have a captive audience. When the stories became too tiresome or if they were bored with them the children would run back into the house. He would then sit on one of the stones on the rockery, mop his brow, sigh, take out his tin of tobacco and slowly roll himself a cigarette. He would light up, and stare malevolently at the two poplars at the bottom of the garden. This pattern never changed: every time he came he followed the same routine. My garden was part of his life, and he came on Wednesday morning at precisely the same time every week. There were times in his story telling when he forgot the childrens' ages and my son still remembers Grandad's horror stories of the blood and muck in the trenches.

I knew Mr Hedge had served in the cavalry, but did not know, until enlightened by my children, that the cavalry in the First World War had also fought in the trenches. My children at times were so fascinated they would ask him questions; he would elaborate, and almost certainly exaggerate to prolong the conversation. He told them he had with his own eyes witnessed soldiers who had gone out of the trenches charging the enemy with bayonets fixed, having their heads shot off. Their bodies however, rifles in their arms, bayonets fixed, continued to charge the enemy. I was pestered by my children to explain this phenomenon, but my explanation of the behaviour of a decerebrate animal which one learns when studying biology in school was too difficult to explain to children of such tender years. They preferred to believe in the supernatural. What amazed me was their lack of anxiety or fright over most of these horror stories. I believe these happenings appeared to be to them in the realms of nursery rhymes – Three Blind Mice, Jack and Jill, Humpty Dumpty – where violence is the norm.

What really plagued Grandad were the two poplars which grew on either side of my back garden and which shaded it. They were so tall that he would moan and grumble about their size. He was old, so were they. As he could not attempt to cut them down he could only stand and hate, while they rustled their branches in mockery. He cursed and cursed and one day one of his curses found its mark; the trees were attacked by a mushroom-type growth which eventually killed them. When he found they had been attacked, his joy was unbounded; it was as if he had won some famous victory over the trees.

When Grandma Hedge died Grandad was in his early eighties, but as he was still a robust fellow he continued as our gardener. Now at least he did not have the poplars to blight his life. Nevertheless, whenever he went into the garden he first looked at the back to see whether some evil spirit had resurrected his enemy. He always carried out the same routine: before pottering about, with his eyes focused on the back brick wall, sat down on one of the stones in the rockery and pensively smoked a cigarette.

Within a few months of his wife's demise he developed a cough, and I sent him for a chest X-ray. This showed a neoplastic growth; in view of his age I decided not to tell him the diagnosis, to say nothing to him, and allow him to work as normal. I did tell the family the diagnosis but my advice to them was that as intensive investigations would not provide a cure, the best thing was to leave him to do my garden and have him X-rayed at intervals afterwards.

Six years after the growth had been found the radiologist who had reported on the first X-ray examination noted that the growth had only marginally increased in size. Grandad told me he had never felt better in his life. He still smoked, still coughed, but had never felt well whilst the poplars stood there. His cough was due to them: not having to work in the shade under those accursed poplars had made all the difference to his health. He would never have had to be X-rayed if they hadn't been there, it was all their fault. I never argued, just agreed. After all, as he was fond of telling me, he came from Somerset: they knew of such goings on there.

Grandad lived until he was nearly ninety; he then had a stroke and departed this life.

6

More Army Tales

Albert Law has been my patient for over thirty years, but it is only in the past few years that he has been complaining of pain in his hips and spine when playing golf. From his life history it is surprising that he has not suffered earlier from these symptoms.

He was born on 14 August 1919 in Avondale Rise, Peckham, went to Bellenden Road School, and on leaving school worked as a printing machine minder. He was called up for National Service on 15 November 1939 and as Rifleman Albert Law, Army No. 6847452, was posted to King's Royal Rifle Corps, stationed in Winchester. After the usual period of square-bashing he was posted to Chiseldon in Wiltshire. In February 1940 he was transferred to the 1st Battalion Queen Victoria Rifles, which was a motorcycle battalion. This battalion spent its time each day playing games, charging around the countryside on mock defence against enemy attacks.

The war began in earnest for Albert, when in the early morning of 22 May 1940, his battalion was sent by train to Dover, minus their vehicles. They boarded the ferry *Canterbury Belle*, and found themselves in Calais one hour later. There were no dockers working in Calais at that time, and they were forced to spend the next five hours unloading their own equipment. Fully equipped with guns and ammunition, but no transport, his platoon was marched five to six miles to a position on the outskirts of Calais.

The German *blitzkrieg* having already broken the back of the French and Allied resistance was now heading straight for the French Channel ports. His battalion however had no idea the enemy was so close. They did not have long to wait! They were soon acquainted of this fact: on the very next morning they found themselves in action against two German armoured divisions who had Calais surrounded.

The front page of one of the morning papers of 22 May 1940 reads: 'A bulge in the German line'.

It must have been referring to his battalion. Some bulge!

They had no chance at all of holding the Germans. Shelled continuously day and night, outgunned, strafed by the Luftwaffe, his battalion still managed to fight its way back into Calais. From the time they had landed in France, they had suffered four days of hell! On the Sunday morning of 26 May 1940, with no food, no water and no more ammunition, they had only one alternative - surrender.

Then began the long march to a German prison camp, via France, Belgium and Holland. For the first two days and nights they were force-marched, without food, water or rest. The fine weather which they had previously enjoyed now gave way to hours of pouring rain. Exhausted, aching all over, bedraggled, now no longer marching but staggering, they were herded as it was getting dark on the third day, into a field, to rest. They just could not have gone on any further. Soldiers were dropping by the roadside, were having to be helped by comrades who were themselves at the end of their tether.

Albert thought himself fortunate in this field; unlike most of his comrades he had retained his gas cape. This had a hood which, with the cape covered him completely, and gave him protection against the elements. Unfortunately, a German soldier saw the cape and ordered Albert to give it to him. He had no alternative, he did so.

As he relates the episode, 'You don't argue with a soldier who has a gun pointed at your chest, and from the look in his eyes is prepared to use it.'

The field was full of puddles of water; it made no difference, they were so exhausted they laid down in it. Suffering from cramp, soaked to the skin, they fell asleep, the sleep of the dead. When they awoke it was daylight: the sun was shining; steam was rising from them as their clothes dried from the heat. To everyone's surprise no one later caught a cold.

The next few weeks were spent in marching back along the same route which the Germans had taken in their advance in to France. They were marched all day, slept rough in the fields at night, and were fed very infrequently. Often as they were marched through French villages women would stand at the door of their houses and throw food to them. There was then a mad scramble by the prisoners to get something to eat. They were starving, the veneer of civilization had left them, they behaved like wild animals, they actually fought one another for scraps of food.

After endless weeks of marching they finally reached the German border. There they were entrained, fifty men per horse wagon, and issued with a small piece of bread and a dab of margarine: this was to last them for a two day journey, to Stalag VIIIB, in Lamsdorf, Upper Silesia.

They had now been eight weeks without a change of clothing, washing facilities of the most primitive type, what more natural than they should all have body lice? Finally arrived in Stalag VIIIB, they stripped off as quickly as they could, washed their clothes and laid them on the ground to dry. They were now in a real prisoner-of-war camp, and while their clothes dried a German barber shaved the prisoners' heads. Albert had not been able to shave since Calais and had by this time grown a Ronald Coleman moustache and long black beard. The German barber who shaved his head was meticulous not to touch his moustache or beard: in this condition he was given a prisoner-of-war number to hold against his chest and a photograph taken.

Should he ever have escaped, the Germans would have been looking for a scraggy, bald-headed old man, with a Charlie Chan moustache and beard. On that day, any view he might have had of German thoroughness, of them being the Master Race, disappeared.

In the prisoner-of-war camp one miserable day was followed by another miserable day. Nights were no better. Depression was the norm: the scanty news which was leaked to them made them even more miserable. The rations were minimal. They were always hungry. One cup of soup each, and two small loaves between nine men was their daily ration. In this condition, while they were so pitifully weak, the Germans began to send out working parties. They were in no fit state to work, but had no choice. He was sent with a party of thirty-five men to maintain railway tracks near pitheads and to dig canals. Silesia was rich in coal mines; there was no shortage of work.

When in a working party, the prisoners did not live in the prisoner-of-war camp but in a bug-ridden house near the coal mine. They were made to parade every morning for work, even those who reported sick were forced to do so by the guard sergeant. The guard sergeant accepted no excuses; you worked until you dropped.

A special day in Rifleman Law's life was 14 August 1940. He remembers it to this day: it was his twenty-first birthday. Through an interpreter he asked for a day off work to celebrate this occasion. Everyone thought his request was outrageous, even the German guards thought he must be mad to make such a request. His audacity however paid off, he got his day off – a rest from ten hours of hard labour.

The winter of 1940 set in. It was freezing cold, dark, depressing, without news from home, without hope. There was twenty to thirty degrees of frost and they were made to work in unbearable conditions. One of the jobs of their working party was to level buckled railway lines. After jacking up a sleeper they had to pack stones underneath. The German overseer as he passed from one working party to the next would shout in broken English, 'No ice under! No ice under!'

After the overseer had passed they would pack as much ice as they could underneath, but were careful to make the track look nice and level. Their work looked good, passed scrutiny, until the thaw set in and the ice melted. The track then looked like a scenic railway, it behaved like one too. Many a derailment took place as a result of their expert workmanship.

One day just before Christmas in 1940 they were issued with a tin of condensed milk, one to each man. On the following day thirty-five packets of tea arrived, to be followed in the next few days by Red Cross parcels. After this they were issued with one Red Cross parcel per man per week. They now felt they were living in luxury!

They still had their lice but had got used to living with them. All their efforts with delousing sessions and steam heating of their clothes had produced no results. Nothing helped. Within a couple of weeks of the Red Cross parcels arriving, the lice simply disappeared. The prisoners were now having more nourishment and came to the conclusion that lice only thrive on undernourished bodies.

In the spring of 1941 they were sent to a coal-mining camp, and Albert spent the next four years working in various mines. One day was spent working in the heat of the coal face, the next, in constant dripping water. The work always alternated in this fashion; it would have taxed the strength of normal healthy men, but the Germans being short of manpower used every individual who could stand on two feet for this back-breaking labour.

In the spring of 1942 he was transferred from a mine in Silesia to a mine in Poland where he found the conditions were a little better. The Poles, also under occupation, worked at a much slower pace and would only do the minimum necessary to keep the Germans happy.

In the pit in which he worked they used cart-horses to bring the coal wagons in and out of the sections from the main thoroughfare. Their section had a long winding track in it, with a drainage ditch about two feet deep on either side. One day, the Germans sent some captured Russian horses to work in this section, Albert's job was to walk alongside them holding the harnesses, teaching them Polish commands: 'Stop! Go! Left! Right!' in Polish.

The horses, who only understood Russian commands, were terrified. Poor Albert was ignored. When the track curved to the right, they turned left. Albert ended up in the drainage ditch. When the track curved to the left, they turned right; he was shoved into the ditch on the opposite side. He now reminisces about what a game it was an Englishman, trying to teach Polish commands to Russian horses!

In the summer of 1944, while still working in a Polish coal-mine in Sosnowiec, near Katowice, his friend suggested they join four other prisoners who were planning an escape. Even if the escape would not be completely successful, a few days of freedom from the drudgery of coal-mining would be a joy. An ingenious plan was devised by one of the prisoners who had by chance discovered the separate tunnel which brought the air pipes down to the pit face. This tunnel was two miles long, with a gradient of one in ten, but still wide enough to be safely negotiated by a prisoner.

When the prisoners went down into the pit each day to work, each one was issued with a metal identity disc, in case of accidents. At the end of the shift, the prisoners remained in the pit until the relieving shift came down. They were then taken up to the surface. On the surface, they dropped their discs in a box provided for the purpose: the guards counted the discs: fifty men had gone down, fifty discs in the box - all OK.

Their escape was planned: he, and five men who were to escape that day, went down on the night shift. They gave their discs to a fellow prisoner on their shift, and he kept the discs until the shift ended. The fellow prisoner went up with seven discs. When the guards counted the discs, fifty men had gone down, fifty discs had been returned - all OK. In the meantime, Albert, and his five fellow escapees, had climbed through the air tunnel into the night air; miles away from the mine. They were free!

This escape had worked so well other men decided to join, just to have a day off. They gave their discs to a chap on their shift, who passed on the discs to a chap on the next shift. They always made sure the number who went down always tallied with the number of discs returned.

Unfortunately, this ruse was discovered after only three days, a stupid prisoner absent-mindedly threw the discs in the box under the watchful eye of the guard. The guard saw one man, why seven discs? He checked and reported the incident. A roll was called, six men were found to be missing. It took many hours and roll calls before the escapees were identified, and the man who put the discs into the box was sentenced to twenty-one days in the 'cooler'.

When Albert and the five other escapees had reached the surface they had immediately walked a few miles in the darkness to get away from the area, before resting in a wood. They then split up into pairs.

He and his partner had made no plan, but thought it would be best if they headed back to Germany where they believed there would be fewer police on the streets. They were wearing the trousers and jackets issued by the Germans for pit work, except the K.G. *(Kriegs Gefarganer)* on the backs of their jackets had been blacked out with shoe polish. They had managed to get hold of a couple of old caps; these they believed would enable them to pretend to be civilian labourers.

For food they had brought with them chocolate, porridge, cocoa, condensed milk and some bread. When the bread ran out they knew they could get no more. Besides being rationed, it would hardly have been wise to go to a shop which sold this commodity and ask for it. Water was their biggest problem. They just could not go to the nearest house to ask for some, they did not know whether the local population would be prepared to risk their necks to help escaping prisoners. They were forced to use streams for drinking water, and in the end it was this problem which led to their recapture. They always slept in a wood at night and walked right through the day until it got dark.

One evening, as usual, they skirted a small town, and bedded down in a copse after drinking from a small stream. They always avoided the big towns because they would have been noticeable; young men in the large towns were conspicuous by their absence. The young men were all doing some form of army service.

After a short time in this copse they were both struck down with diarrhoea which continued right through the night. The morning found them cold, tired, bad tempered and exhausted. At midday, they decided to move and after walking a few miles threw caution to the wind. Instead of skirting a small town they walked right through it. They were so fed up they began to quarrel, blamed each other for their predicament, did not care who heard them. They were squabbling in English, people passing by gave them startled looks, and quickly hurried away. Living in a police state, no one wanted to get involved with the authorities, even to the extent of reporting suspicious characters.

They walked right through the town, back into the countryside, shouting at each other, until they were exhausted. They then sat down to rest on the side of a cornfield. The cornfield was next to a road, and along this road came a policeman nonchalantly riding his bicycle. He stopped when he saw them. He was over fifty years of age, five foot nothing in height, sported a small moustache and wore thick spectacles. He asked for their identity papers.

They had by this time had enough of freedom; they explained to him in their best German that they were escaped prisoners-of-war. He became wild with excitement, almost kissed them in his frenzy, nothing like this had ever happened to him. He ordered Albert's friend to wheel his bicycle for him while he walked behind them pointing his rifle at their backs. He led them to the police station. He was so happy, he told everyone who passed, singlehandedly, he had captured '*Zwei Englander*'.

The police station to which they were taken was a tiny, old, ramshackle country place, manned by a sergeant who appeared even older than the policeman who had effected their capture. The sergeant too became excited when he realized who they were, locked them in a cell, and gave them some bread and ersatz coffee. At that particular moment the food tasted delicious! The sergeant telephoned the camp from which they had escaped; he was told the prisoners would have to spend a night in the cell and a guard from the camp would come and collect them in the morning.

Their cell though small was rather strange; there were no bars in the window. After bread and coffee Albert felt much more comfortable, looked down out of the 'barless' cell window to see what lay below. Looking up at him was a huge hungry looking Alsatian dog sitting on the grass outside, wagging its tail, daring him to try it!

The camp guard arrived the next morning and they were taken by local train back to their prisoner-of-war camp. On the train was a group of Waffen SS who, when they found out who the prisoners were, gave them a chorus of the song 'Marching against England'. There was however no animosity; the SS after a lusty rendering of their party piece came over to them, and chatted about the Russian front; they even gave them cigarettes.

On their arrival back at the prisoner-of-war camp they were sentenced to five days in a German military prison and learned there that of the six prisoners who had made the initial escape, two more had been recaptured, but two had made it. They knew that the two who had made good their escape, instead of making for Germany intended to go to Warsaw. They later learned that these two had actually got to Warsaw, and had taken part in the uprising.

A few weeks after their recapture, there was a statement read on parade which put an end to any more attempts. This statement read: 'Escaping is no longer a sport. In future, escaping prisoners caught wearing civilian clothes will be shot as spies.'

No one attempted to escape after this warning; it was just not worth it. There was no doubt in any of the prisoners' minds that the Germans would carry out their threat. After all, the Germans could legitimately claim prisoners-of-war had to be in uniform to be granted the privilege of being called prisoners, not spies.

That summer, in 1944, as their day shift ambled through the main gate into the compound, they saw an Aussie prisoner-of-war lying on a blanket in a pair of shorts, sunbathing. His left arm was sticking up in the air from a flexed elbow, whilst his index finger was heavily bandaged.

'What happened to you?' he was asked by his friend who happened to be one of the workers on Albert's shift.

'Broke my finger,' he replied. 'A chunk of stone fell and crushed my finger on the rim of a skip I was pushing.'

'You lucky sod!' said his friend. 'Is dinner ready?'

'All laid on,' he said, getting to his feet.

On the following day, as the shift came into their compound after the day's work, they saw two Aussies sunbathing. Now two fingers pointed to the sky.

'It must be contagious,' someone in their group shouted.

The next day, four bodies were sunbathing, four

heavily bandaged fingers pointed to the sky: elbows flexed, resting neatly on blankets, completed the scene.

'You bloody Aussies must have a bone deficiency,' someone shouted.

'Something funny going on,' said Albert's friend.

'Lucky buggers!' Albert thought.

Later that night they were awakened by the sound of a terrible scream, they shot out of bed and ran to the room from where the scream emanated. All the occupants of the room were gathered round one bed. The man in the bed was sitting up in bed, wringing his left hand, moaning.

'Nothing to worry about,' said the Aussie prisoners round the man's bed.

'Jack wanted Dr Hartley to do his finger, but couldn't face it in cold blood, so arranged to have it done while asleep.'

Dr Hartley was an Australian from the Outback, nicknamed 'Doc' by the Aussies for his work on producing 'bathing beauties', whose fingers pointed to the sky – the envy of every shift who returned from a sweaty day on the coal face. When he was asked how he did it he drawled, 'I take a strip of blanket, one layer on the edge of the bunk, then place the finger on it. Another layer on top of the finger, short sharp whack with my iron bar, and the job's done!'

The patient after this operation would report for work normally on the following day, but after a reasonable time would report an 'accident' to the overseer. Under the safety regulations this had to be done, no one was going to break the regulations!

There were ten broken fingers in six days, the Germans became suspicious. They could not understand nor could they account for the way the accidents had occurred. They knew the fingers were definitely broken, and all in the mine, but the number of accidents was well above the normal.

By the seventh morning the Germans had had enough; all the sick were transported to the nearest military hospital to be examined by German doctors. Albert too was taken, he had been absent from work for a few days because of a skin complaint. After being examined the only ten men passed fit for work by the German doctors were the ten with the broken fingers. The Germans had evidently solved the mystery and knew the cause.

Early in 1945, the Russian offensive which had been initiated on 12 January, began advancing towards the mine in which Albert worked. The great 'Winter March' for the prisoners-of-war began.

With a little Red Cross food they left the mine and were marched westward, through Poland, Czechoslovakia, up and down the Bavarian Alps to South-West Germany. It was freezing cold. At night they were forced to sleep in barns. They were awakened at dawn, and marched until it got too dark to see. Marching over the Bavarian Alps was no joke. It snowed a lot of the time; they were starving, and frozen to the marrow. To add to their discomfiture they kept slipping and sliding over packed snow in the mountain passes.

One evening they saw prisoners from a concentration camp being marched in front of them. These other prisoners were gaunt and thin, like corpses, they could not believe their eyes: these prisoners were in an even worse condition than they were themselves. They marched on and suddenly came across a body lying on the side of the road, shot in the forehead. It was one of the concentration camp marchers. The wound had not bled, it was too cold! They passed several more bodies frozen in the moment of death, in grotesque positions. With the war obviously coming to an end they could not understand why the Germans continued to kill, just for the fun of it. Their own guards had always treated them humanely; they had not realized that the German guards in charge of concentration camp prisoners had become so dehumanized that their prisoners had become no better than animals in their eyes.

One night the barn in which they would have to sleep led through a farmyard, and they noticed a big clump of potatoes in the corner. The potatoes were there for just five minutes! When the farmer discovered his loss the guard commander searched them, but by that time the prisoners had them well-hidden in the straw. When the coast was clear, they were taken out and eaten - raw.

On another occasion they were put in a barn where there were chickens pecking at food in the farmyard. An Aussie prisoner had previously shown them how to put a chicken's head under its wing, rock it a few times so it stayed still, and the bird then appeared to be asleep. These chickens in the farmyard disappeared! Another parade, another search. The farmer's wife was crying, the guards were ranting and raving, all to no avail! The prisoners denied taking chickens, when out of the barn staggered a half-plucked chicken, which had not been properly put to sleep the Aussie way. The guards went mad, the prisoners were threatened with all sorts of punishment, but they were at the end of their tether, they didn't care any more. No punishment however was meted out to them, the guards themselves had by this time realized it would have been to their own disadvantage to do so. The guards had communication with the outside, knew the situation at the battle fronts, were now only interested in saving their own skins.

They were marched on, after three months they had reached an area near Regensburg. One morning they awoke to find that their guards had deserted them. They had disarmed themselves, neatly stacked their rifles, and were waiting to be taken prisoner themselves. The Yanks were coming. They were free!

The prisoners now free, left to their own devices, wandered into the nearest village, and billeted themselves in various houses. The houses in the village were mainly occupied by women, the men having long been taken away for army service. No one in the village refused to accept their new lodgers; the occupants really had no choice, it paid them to be nice to their new visitors.

The Yanks came through in their tanks later on that day, realized immediately who these bedraggled men were by their uniforms, and threw food and cigarettes from their tanks to them. They were then left to fend for themselves, and stood at the side of the road during the daylight hours watching the Yanks go by. All sorts of gifts were thrown to them by these 'liberators'.

After a couple of weeks of Yank-watching, of recuperation, as no one appeared to be interested in them, after all the war for them had ended, Albert, with some other ex-prisoners managed to hitch a lift in an American transporter which was going to an army base camp. In this camp they were interrogated to make sure they really were British, then flown home in a Lancaster bomber which was on a routine flight bringing in supplies.

How he survived those five long years as a prisoner-of-war he will never know.

What for?

So that he can now plague me with his symptoms of arthritis for which I have no cure.

Mr Sharples walked into my consulting rooms one day, saw my army group photograph which is on the wall, looked at me and said, 'Boyce Barracks, Crookham.'

This photograph had been taken in 1948, when I first joined the army during my six weeks' square bashing, and I asked how he knew. He said he recognized some of the officers in the photograph, he himself had been posted there in late October 1946. Being a fellow comrade, I now asked him how he had come to be in my regiment, he then gave me his life history.

He was born in 1928, in Wolstanton, a village in North Staffordshire. After he left school, having difficulty in finding a suitable job in the area, he decided to come to London where work could more easily be found. Work was not all that easy to find even in London, so he was not disappointed to be called up for army service in October 1946.

Private Sharples, Army No. 19090789, did his basic training at Maidstone with the Royal West Kent Regiment, then applied and was accepted after an examination, for the Royal Army Medical Corps. He did six weeks basic training in Crookham, where I had been stationed, where the photograph had been taken, and while there had volunteered for duty in Palestine.

He sailed from Liverpool in January 1947, but the boat instead of going straight to Palestine docked first at Port Said, in Egypt. From Port Said he was transferred to the base depot at El Ballah, then posted to the British Military Hospital in Haifa.

The one journey in his life he will never forget and constantly reminds me of, is the one from El Kantara in Egypt, to Haifa in Palestine. He was in an army train, and the perfume of the orange blossom on crossing the border from Sinai into Palestine was so heady as to be intoxicating. The novelty of children tossing huge Jaffa oranges into their train as it passed through Gaza was exciting too.

The British Military Hospital in Haifa had belonged to the Italian monks before the British took over, but in their possession had only been a small building with a hundred beds. This had been much too small for the British requirements and they had built on. By the time Private Sharples arrived the hospital had increased in size to hold 400 beds. Extra medical and surgical wards had been added. Some of the wards were housed in Nissen huts in the hospital grounds, the remainder in a compound adjacent to the main building. The main building itself housed the operating theatre and support departments. These included dispensary, blood bank, X-ray and dental department. The rest of the building was divided into offices and other ranks' surgical wards.

The compound adjacent to the main building contained the medical wards, pathology laboratory, staff (other rank billets), quartermaster stores and NAAFI. It also contained a cinema, which doubled as a theatre. As the mortuary was already at that time inadequate for their needs it only had one slab, a much larger one was built in the grounds - at a distance from the main building.

Shortly after he arrived, the Irgun (Israeli Freedom Fighters) blew up the Iraqi Petroleum Company's refinery in the Port area. It had obviously been done for his benefit, to acclimatize him to the conflict! This was early in 1947.

Immediately after this a police station at Kingsway was attacked and there were many casualties. These casualties were civil police and did not come to the British Military Hospital, but went to the Government Hospital in the Lower Port area at Kyat instead. The attack on the police station had been made by a catapult machine mounted on the back of a canvas-covered van.

The missile, an oil drum packed with explosives with an impact detonator, had scored a direct hit on the station. It had been propelled up a ramp. By this means it had been shot high in the air which had enabled it to clear the ten foot high security fence. It had landed against the wall of the police station, blowing out the front of the building.

His version of the attack by the Irgun on 4 May 1947 against the crusader fortress at Acre, which was being used by the British as a prison, was that it was timed to be carried out when the prisoners were on afternoon exercise. This fortress, when in Ottoman hands, had successfully withstood a siege by Napoleon's forces in 1799 and it was no mean feat which the Irgun was attempting. Some explosives had been smuggled in beforehand with the object of releasing some Irgun prisoners held in the jail by demolishing part of the prison wall from the inside.

The Irgun assault on the fortress had been a finely coordinated operation, and some thirty Irgun men, a number of members of the Stern gang, and many Arab prisoners managed to escape. A group of British soldiers in the vicinity engaged the Irgun, and in the ensuing battle nine Irgun men were killed.

Pte Sharples had been rushed to the scene from base hospital with a six ambulance accompaniment, but there was little they could do; most of the casualties were dead. He remembers clearly the event. After the last of our ambulances had crossed the open country which led to Acre, the road behind them had been blown up by the Irgun: there were many casualties in this incident too.

The common jargon in their mess was, 'If your number is on the bloody missile, there is no escape.'

One poor young lad had both his feet blown off having just arrived in Haifa. His number had been on that missile.

A major in the Royal Army Service Corps had been brought into the hospital one day with an impacted fracture of the skull. Fortunately for him at the time there was only superficial brain damage, the skull fragments were removed and the space packed. Later, the dental technician made a plate which was sutured into the skull and when the hair was combed back the scar was invisible. They were all delighted! Unfortunately they had forgotten their mess jargon. The major's number had really been on the original missile, but either in its trajectory the missile had lost its aim or had forgotten his number, the major had recovered. Two weeks later another missile did not make the same mistake, the major was shot in the chest and died in transit. Incidentally, the plate in the major's skull was removed at the post mortem.

On numerous occasions they were called in the middle of the night to help unload and transport injured Jewish immigrants from Royal Navy ships who had intercepted immigrant ships while they were trying to enter Palestine illegally. He and his friends always felt sorry for the poor devils who had suffered unimaginable trials and tribulations in German concentration camps, only to be apprehended within sight of their 'Promised Land'. Amongst the ships he saw escorted into Haifa was the ship featured in the book *Exodus* by Leon Uris. The ships carrying the refugees were often dilapidated junkyard boats of all sizes and shapes, most of them not fit to be on the Thames, never mind a sea journey. When apprehended by the navy they were escorted into Haifa and tied up in the harbour facing the hospital cinema. They were a constant reminder to the hospital staff of man's inhumanity to man.

As soon as the water melons came into season the hospital wards filled up. There were widespread epidemics of typhoid fever whilst he was in Haifa and they were also hit by an epidemic of cholera brought in from Egypt. On one occasion they even had an attack of bubonic plague. Whenever an epidemic was prevalent the cinema was closed, and all the troops in North Palestine were brought in for inoculation.

When Palestine was finally partitioned by the United Nations on 24 November 1947, Pte Sharples and the rest of the troops breathed a sigh of relief. They were not politicians; they thought that peace would reign. No such luck. The Jews and the Arabs, instead of fighting the British now fought each other. Jewish buses and cars were now covered with armour and all the seats, except those of the drivers, were removed.

The boundary fence of the medical compound of the hospital bordered the Tel Aviv to Haifa road, and on the other side of the road from the compound was an Arab garage. The British knew that this garage specialized in making armoured cars to attack the Egged buses (Jewish) which used the road, but did nothing about it. The Jews however were determined to keep this main road open at all costs, and one night they attacked the garage with hand-grenades and a Piat anti-tank gun. Though the battle was on their doorstep the British did not interfere, but the noise gave them all a very sleepless night.

A few months before the British pulled out of Palestine, Pte Sharples was faced with his own problems. He spilled iodine all down the front of his overall by dropping a demi-john. This demi-john knocked over a primus in his dispensary igniting the iodine, and poor Sharples sustained second degree burns to his left leg. He now became a hospital patient himself for a few weeks, and as he could not stand for long periods he was transferred from the dispensary to the pathology laboratory. His arrival at the laboratory was fortuitous; it coincided with an outbreak of typhoid fever, and his first job was to take samples from the patients' overnight bedpans.

He was delighted when he was told that he was being demobilized and returned to the UK, but not so happy that he was first going to be sent back to the British Military Hospital at El-Ballah in Egypt. From El-Ballah, he was transferred to a British Military Hospital in Malta, then to England, on the good ship *Empress of Australia,* in February 1949. At the time, he was glad to see the back of Palestine, but has often expressed the wish to return, now that stability has returned to that country. He has no animosity: only respect for what the Jews have achieved in such a short period of time.

7

Naughty, Naughty!

In 1970, I was called out one Saturday afternoon whilst on rota duty to a very beautiful Jamaican nurse whom I had met previously several times in the surgery. She was a patient of one of my partners, and I had never previously had occasion to treat her.

It was a lovely, hot, June day, when this visit was requested, and as she lived in a flat in Lausanne Road, I could easily walk the distance if I wanted to. On arriving at the flat I was not surprised when she opened the door in her dressing-gown; after all, she was supposed to be ill, and there was no one else to let me in. I was also not surprised when she led me into her bedroom. The surprise came in her subsequent behaviour. She proceeded to undress completely. She took off her dressing-gown, her nightdress, lay naked on the bed, and opened her legs.

'I know what you want,' she said, 'Please get it over and done with quickly.'

I am a coward, perhaps it was her saying 'please', which threw me. I didn't know what to say or how to handle the situation, I grabbed my bag and fled.

She phoned again on Sunday, the following day, requested a visit, and sounded very rational. I answered the phone myself, but she made no apology for the previous day's performance, just said that she needed an injection of Depixol – this is given to psychotic patients in need of therapy. I had not previously known that she was in need of therapy.

I can't explain why but I had the feeling that the previous day's performance on her part was an aberration and not in line with her normal behaviour, so I went to her flat again. Once again she appeared in her dressing-gown, but was completely rational, and made no mention of the previous day: neither did I. I gave her an injection of Depixol and fled, in case she tried to tempt me with her naked body again.

I had no reason to see this nurse again, my partner returned the next day and took over her management.

I learned from him that she was married to a normal chap, who had a hell of a life in coping with her. She gave him so much aggravation that in spite of her beauty he was finally compelled to divorce her.

☆ ☆ ☆

Mr Fredericks (George), a seventy-two year old grey-haired gentleman, came into the surgery one evening in August 1979 as an emergency, to consult me about his 'private' parts. He lived with his mother and brother Joe in Lyndhurst Grove, but although I had treated his mother and brother on many occasions I could not recollect ever having previously seen him. His appearance was so distinctive that I could never have forgotten.

He and his brother were bachelors, had been excellent sons, and had spent their lives looking after the old lady who was in her eighties. There was a married sister in the area too whom I did not know, and from the old lady's description of her I was not missing much. The sister only appeared on high days and holy days and left her mother at all the other times to be cared for by her brothers. This arrangement continued until the old lady died in 1976, the brothers were then left to care for each other. I never heard either brother speak of a sister afterwards; if their mother had never mentioned her, I would not have known there had been a third member of the family.

My first encounter with George occurred three years after his mother's death. He appeared at my surgery wearing a dirty wide trilby hat pulled well down over his forehead, dirty long mackintosh, greasy trousers with turnups, and an old, dirty, crumpled shirt, which looked as if it had never been washed. His shirt collar was open, even though he sported a tie which by its appearances seemed as old as himself. On a peremptory look – his dress personified 'a flasher' – a dirty old man.

He told the receptionists when he appeared at their desk that he was an emergency, needed to see a doctor urgently, but refused to say what was wrong with him. He insisted that he see me, I was his doctor, and I was the one he intended to see however long he waited. The receptionist had no alternative but to fit him in to one of my emergency appointment slots. He was sent to the waiting-room and took his seat in the crowded room without making any fuss. When I opened the door to the waiting-room to call in the next patient, my eyes could not fail to notice this odd looking character, his bashed-up hat firmly ensconced on his head. I must admit I called him in to see me before his appointed time. One reason was curiosity; he did look like a dirty old tramp; the other reason was that he stank out the waiting-room. Patients waiting in the room looked at me appealingly whenever a new patient was ushered in. We both received dirty looks.

When I finally called him in I shook his hand and showed him to a seat. The seat part was something I had debated in my mind before his entrance. He was such an unkempt looking character I thought that when I finally called him in, I should keep him standing! I asked him for his complaints, but he first began to explain why he insisted on only seeing me – he knew me from his Mom. He told me he had been a porter in Covent Garden vegetable market all his life, and never previously been ill. He had been registered with me for over twenty-five years, and had never troubled me.

Mr Fredericks had never had time to be ill, apart from a weekly visit to the West End had spent all his time and money on his old Mom. It was obvious from his first few remarks that he had worshipped her, and the care lavished on her probably explained why she was almost ninety when she died.

We now spent some time speaking about his old Mom for I remembered her well. She had been a tiny shrivelled up old lady, almost bent double by her arthritis, who shuffled slowly to the front door to open it. Her living-room had been in the back of the house and a visit to her had always taken up a lot of my time.

George was friendly and communicative. Although we had never previously met, he had obviously heard a lot about me from his old Mom. I was however running late, also out of patience, and asked him what the real reason for his trip to me was. He didn't answer. He stood up, peeled off his dirty mackintosh, took off a threadbare coat jacket, unbuttoned the fly buttons of his trousers, and produced to my startled gaze – his penis. One thing he did not remove was his hat, which remained firmly planted on his head. For this I was grateful, to gaze on the jungle which lay under this canopy was something I feared. He had not said a word whilst this unbuttoning was taking place. To be perfectly honest, I had not paid much attention when he was unveiling, I had been reading a letter from a hospital consultant relating to some accident which this fellow had suffered as a young boy.

George was the first to break the ice. 'Will you have a look at my dick? I think I have got VD,' he said.

I looked at him in amazement. He explained, because his penis had irritated him on the previous day he had examined it and to his horror had found a rash. My retort was, 'It is impossible. How can you think of such a thing? You don't get VD from a lavatory seat, you should know better than that. Let me have a look. What makes you think that you have got VD?'

Without the slightest embarrassment, he gave me a history of going regularly once a week to a French prostitute in the West End. Why he insisted on saying that she was French I never asked.

He had been going to the same one and only lady for twenty-five years. She was now in her fifties. When on the very few occasions she had not been available, when she was on holiday for instance, she had provided him with a young French girl. He told me all this while still standing in front of me almost naked. He was certainly a sight to behold: a hat perched on his head, the brim of which almost covered his eyes, shirt pulled up to his neck, and trousers down to his ankles. His dirty well-worn underpants, which had not seen the sight of soap and water for many months, hovered midway between his buttocks and feet.

He suddenly stopped and thought.

'I've got it,' he said, 'it's the young girl, she's the culprit, she's the last one I went with!'

He explained that the young girl, in her early twenties, had been trained by Madam, so he could not really understand how he could have caught anything. Still, she was the last one! The ladies were meticulously clean and hygienic, had always washed him down thoroughly themselves before allowing him to perform. From his appearance as he stood before me, I was not surprised!

In the early years, when he had first made use of the 'lady's' services she had charged him two pounds.

'It was a lot of money in those days,' he said.

As the years had passed she had been forced to increase her prices, and two months ago she had increased them once again. It was now twelve pounds and even this rate was a special one as he was a regular customer and an old age pensioner.

One thing he would not do, however hard I tried, was to tell me the exact address of his 'lady'. He would only say that she advertised her services in the press as a model, and provided massage services both in her premises and in clients' homes. Her premises from which she worked was a flat over a shop in the Leicester Square area and he had a regular appointment there.

His appointment was every Wednesday afternoon at 2.30 p.m. – this time had been the same since he retired. He had come to see me on Tuesday, and he had an appointment for the following day which he had no wish to cancel; this is why he had insisted on seeing me as an emergency. When he had been at work he had not been able to go during the week and his appointment then had been on Saturday afternoon at 4.30 p.m. He had always been allowed exactly three quarters of an hour of her time, then politely shown the door marked 'exit'. Why he specifically mentioned an exit sign on her door I did not have the temerity to ask.

Because of the journey, he was now always given a cup of tea and a biscuit on his arrival. He had only subscribed to this one lady and was now treated more or less as a member of her family.

I asked how he managed to get to the West End.

'Why, I use my bus pass,' he said.

I had long since lost my irritation at the time I was taking in seeing Mr Fredericks for I was enjoying his narrative. I had already been in practice for twenty-seven years and had never met such a colourful character.

After giving me such a long history I felt duty bound to examine him thoroughly, and he was delighted to hear that he had not contracted a venereal disease. His ladies had behaved impeccably and they could have had no influence on the diagnosis. The rash on his penis was due to thrush. Urine and blood examinations later confirmed it was due to diabetes. I treated him successfully for this complaint until 1991, when he suddenly went into heart failure and departed this life. Whether he went back to his lady to celebrate after I had made the initial diagnosis, I never had the courage to ask!

One Saturday night, or rather early Sunday morning, in January 1968 whilst on rota duty, I was asked to visit a patient who was not registered with me, but was a patient of one of the rota doctors. The request made to my wife on the telephone was for me to visit a child suffering from earache in a block of flats opposite St Giles's Hospital. Although St Giles's Hospital is within walking distance of my surgery, it was not from my home at the time in Brockley; it was three miles away.

It was 2.30 a.m., I had been woken from my sleep, I

was not feeling in the best of moods. To add to my irritability, to my discomfort, it was a cold, rainy, miserable, dark night. The temperature hovered at the freezing point level, the trees in Hillyfields park opposite appeared to be trying to keep themselves warm, as their branches completely naked violently shook in the wind.

As my wife had been informed by the patient's mother the child had already been allowed to suffer the pain for a couple of days, also as this patient was not one of mine, I was feeling quite depressed at having to get out of bed. At that moment, I hated the National Health Service, its demand that I work unsocial hours, and its lack of understanding in failing to reward me for doing so.

My car must have felt my mood: not wishing to add to my distress, it gave me no trouble at all in starting: in spite of the cold and damp it started immediately. There was little traffic on the road so in no time at all I was able to park my car outside the flats.

I was met at the entrance by a smart, well-dressed, short-skirted, heavily made-up girl in her late teens, whom I assumed had come to meet me to take me to the patient. I had noted these particulars of the girl in a flash for she was very attractive, but I thought her face would have benefited by not being so heavily plastered with make-up.

I was not surprised at her being at the entrance of the block to meet me. On night duty it was not unusual for a member of the patient's family to be waiting anxiously outside to escort me to their residence. On many occasions when on a home confinement I had been almost dragged from my car by an anxious husband in an hysterical condition. I also remember the time when as soon as my car had stopped, a husband had opened my door, grabbed my case and ran, knowing full well that

I would not be far behind.

The number of the flat I was visiting on this Sunday morning was nineteen. I had no problem following this relative from the cheap perfume she was using and the clonk clonk of her stiletto heels on the concrete stairs. Her perfume, as was obviously intended, wafted behind her in the enclosed corridors of the block; it was supposed to be intoxicating; it made me want to vomit.

The block I was visiting was an old one with a winding staircase. As the landings were very dark, the sound of the young lady's footsteps was reassuring; I was not being made to search for the flat. The smell of her perfume as it wafted behind her also acted as a guide, and while I could hear the clonking I knew that we had not yet reached our destination. It was after two o'clock in the morning, the last thing I wanted to do was to search for a number in the dark. I was feeling rather grateful to the family for providing me with an escort.

We had reached the fourth floor. Overweight, and carrying a heavy doctor's case full of instruments and drugs, I suddenly felt rather tired and exhausted. My mind cleared. What were we doing on the fourth floor? I had been given nineteen as the number of the flat by my wife. I stopped to check the note on which the visit had been written. It was nineteen. My escort however was still climbing the stairs. In my mind I thought, surely nineteen could not be higher than the fourth floor? I flashed my torch, and its light illuminated the number plate on the door of the flat to my right, on this landing. The number stood out like a beacon; as if it was mocking me. It was thirty-nine. There was definitely something wrong.

The young lady 'relative' had by now almost reached the fifth floor. I ran up the steps and caught up with her.

As I stood next to her, panting after my efforts to catch up, I was almost gassed by the smell of her perfume. She had almost certainly bathed in the stuff, the heavy odour took one's breath away.

'What number are we going to, love?' I asked, my speech coming in short pants from my exertions. She must have thought, when I recollect the incident, this customer is dying for it, he can't wait.

'What's it to you?' she replied.

'I'm the doctor on my way to visit a sick child with earache at number nineteen,' I said.

She stopped. Although it was too dark to see her, there was no mistaking the anger in her voice.

'What the bloody hell do you want to drag me up here for? You're no f...... good to me!' she said.

She roughly brushed past me; I almost fell as she rushed back down the stairs. The stupid girl had picked the wrong customer. I was left to drag myself after her.

Number nineteen was two floors down!

☆ ☆ ☆

When I was working as a rota doctor for a group of doctors in the East End of London in 1954 an incident occurred which I cannot forget, and I still remember it with amusement.

After doing a surgery in my own practice in Peckham, to supplement my income I worked nights as a duty doctor for a group of ten doctors. My duty commenced at seven o'clock in the evening, I never had less than seven visits a night, never got to bed before two o'clock in the morning and slept afterwards at Dr Cyderman's surgery in New Road, off the Commercial Road, in a room over the shop front. I invariably had to start doing the visits at eight o'clock in the evening, and was kept working continuously until after midnight. Not knowing the area, more often than not I got lost on my travels. On returning to base after my last visit I would fall exhausted on to a put-u-up which the elderly housekeeper who had a flat on the top floor had prepared for me. I earned the princely sum of two pounds per night, for being on duty from seven o'clock at night until seven o'clock in the morning.

At three o'clock in the morning, in December 1954, I had been asleep for exactly two hours when the housekeeper came into my room to wake me; to attend to this foreign sailor who had come for private medical attention. This surgery was often used by these gentlemen for their medical requirements. By word of mouth they knew they could receive a penicillin injection for their venereal disease; they often presented themselves for this treatment without suffering from the complaint. Having had sex with a lady who frequented the docks, they thought that prevention by having an injection of penicillin was better than waiting for the disease to show itself.

The sailor, the cause of my awakening, was Portuguese. His English was most rudimentary and I, thirty-seven years after the event, still do not know one word of Portuguese. His English was so bad that it took me a quarter of an hour even to find out which part of his anatomy he was complaining about. I finally got out of him that he could not 'piss'. I then spent a long time questioning him, trying to find out the cause. At three in the morning my English, attempting to get him to understand what I was endeavouring to extract from him in the way of symptoms was not of the best quality. I kept slipping into Yiddish and German thinking this would help, but it only added to the confusion. Somehow, I finally managed to make him understand, I wanted to know how long he had gone without passing water.

He answered, 'Nine hours.'

I naturally assumed he had come with some venereal infection, and with pornographic sign language made him realize I wanted to know when he had last had sex with a woman. His answer was precise, 'Woman four days.'

His face suddenly screwed up with pain. He turned white, broke out in a sweat, and swayed on the chair. I caught him before he fell and half carried, half walked him to the examination couch. I laid him on his back and assisted him in taking his trousers down. My intention was to examine his abdomen for urinary retention. What I saw I could hardly believe. He had a tight constriction in the middle of his penis with the foreskin bulging and swollen. His penis was about three times its normal size and looked likely to burst. This was causing the urinary retention!

On examination I found that the constriction was caused by a curtain ring which had been forced down the middle of the shaft. The curtain ring could not be seen because of the swelling, and I had to forcibly stretch the organ, causing immense pain, before I found out what was causing the obstruction. He broke out in a sweat whilst I was examining him, and I thought he might faint at any moment.

I advised him to go to hospital, but he adamantly refused. I gave him a drink of water whilst he explained to me in broken English that his ship was sailing to Sweden at eight that morning – he had to be on that ship. He cried, begged me to help him so pitifully that I just could not refuse.

With the help of Ethyl Chloride, a local anaesthetic, it took me two hours to cut through the ring and remove it from his male organ. Luckily for me, the doctor's surgery contained a ring cutter. Luckily for him, I had been a casualty officer in the Victoria Hospital, Blackpool, and had cut rings off previously – but only from fingers!

His story, in very broken English which he told me as he relaxed after the successful operation, was that he had been held down by fellow sailors while the ring had been put on. He had tried to remove it himself without success; his efforts had only made matters worse.

'More I try, more ring on prick,' were his actual words.

I did not know whether to believe his story, but the relief on his face after the removal of the ring was a sight to behold. He left in ample time to make it back to his ship; I suppose his refusal to go to hospital was justified.

I can quite understand why sailors from the docks came to this doctor's surgery; the housekeeper never refused entrance to them at any time of the day or night. I learned afterwards that she made a very profitable business from these visits, and encouraged them. She set the charges, and pocketed half of the proceeds for herself. The removal of the ring had cost the Portuguese sailor twenty pounds, an enormous sum of money, a fortune.

I knew I was going to get ten pounds out of it; she always treated me fairly and gave me half of her charges. With my financial state being so perilous at that particular time, I really could not have afforded to turn my back on the 'Lord of the Ring'.

8

Peckham Wry

While driving along Nunhead Lane at 11.30 one morning in April 1966 I was caught in a police speed trap. I had turned left, from Linden Grove into Nunhead Lane, there were no traffic lights at that junction in those days, and I was speeding along nonchalantly towards Peckham Rye when a policeman suddenly appeared in the road. There is a bend in the road at this point, and the policeman appeared as out of thin air on the passenger side, between two parked cars, and ordered me to stop. Being a law-abiding citizen I did as I was requested. I had no choice. I would have knocked him down if I had carried on. He was horrified when he saw me.

'My God,' he said, 'it's the Doctor!'

I didn't recognize him at all, but thought that he had identified me as a doctor from the badge on my windscreen. I learned afterwards that this was not so, he had actually recognized me. He was the husband of the lady I had attended the previous night for the delivery of their child. I had spent a large part of the night attending to his wife, as I had been summoned by the midwives to attend to her as an emergency. She was not a patient of mine, I had never seen the couple before but during the long night he presumably had time to remember my features. He had been present at the birth, but I had been so involved with his wife's confinement I did not remember his face. Besides, the chap who now stopped me was in police uniform, and uniform always appears to alter a person's appearance.

The policeman, PC Jarvis, explained to me that the sergeant who was on duty with him in the speed trap was not in his present mood very friendly to doctors. He would however do his best for me, but would make no promises.

'For God's sake keep quiet, leave it to me and say nothing, Doc.'

I didn't answer, he was acting the perfect policeman, authority with dignity; I hadn't recognized him, so did not understand why he would be so conciliatory in trying to protect me from the dreaded sergeant.

The sergeant, in plain clothes, was walking towards my car but had not yet reached it, when the constable left me to intercept him.

The speed trap 'set up' had been: the sergeant stood at the first checkpoint with a stopwatch, a second policeman stood at a set distance with his stopwatch at the second checkpoint, and PC Jarvis (my policeman as I later discovered) further on. When a motorist exceeded the limit, PC Jarvis's duty was to order him to stop. He had done his duty, having been signalled to do so, had stopped me.

PC Jarvis and the sergeant came up to my car walking together and I could see that the sergeant had a particularly disturbed and thunderous look on his face. As he was in plain clothes, if it had not been for PC Jarvis and the sergeant's 'particular' walk, I would not have known that the sergeant was in the police force. Only people in authority walk in this fashion. Every sergeant major I had encountered during my army service had this gait. This sergeant walked with slow, even, deliberate, intimidating steps, each step exactly the same length, to the inch, as the previous one!

I remained in my driver's seat with the window turned down, while the pair of them conferred, standing in the road, looking down at me. PC Jarvis was explaining to the sergeant that I was a doctor on an urgent visit having spent most of the previous night attending to his wife and having been delayed in the process.

Now I knew why he was trying to shield me! He was so apologetic, his phraseology so servile even I squirmed. The sergeant listened in a pensive fashion, stroked his face and when PC Jarvis had completed his obsequious speech, proceeded to give me a lecture. He put his head through my car window, glared at me for what appeared to be an eternity, then in a restrained voice ordered me to curb my speed in the future in built up areas.

'You're a doctor,' he said, 'I don't suppose you're a bloody fool or the police constable wouldn't have spoken so highly of you. Why when you know the speed limit is thirty miles an hour in built up areas don't you stick to it?'

I just sat there in the driver's seat shamefaced, saying, 'Yes sergeant, no sergeant,' whenever I thought it was judicious to say so.

He ended up by saying very crossly, 'Now don't write to thank me for not booking you!'

This last statement foxed me. I did not understand what he meant, but thought it prudent to sit silent. He then waved me on, and I did not hesitate to drive away at the fastest permissible speed. I had forgotten all about the incident until I went to see PC Jarvis's wife that evening and her husband was at home to let me in. He explained I had been extremely lucky at not being summoned for a speeding offence that day. Even he did not think he could have persuaded the sergeant to let me go with a caution.

It appeared an Indian doctor had a similar incident, driving over the speed limit three weeks previously and the sergeant, always merciful to doctors, had sent him away with a caution. The doctor had then written a thank you letter to the superintendent at the police station praising the sergeant.

The doctor in his letter praised the sergeant who had been in plain clothes, the two policemen in uniform, the Queen for being the head of such a wonderful nation, the government who had such a fine body of men to protect the country, and the quality and professionalism of the British police for only cautioning him for a speeding offence. The one person whom he had forgotten to thank was the superintendent, but it would not have made the slightest difference.

The sergeant had got a rocket from the superintendent reminding him that he was not the chief of police. He was not even a superintendent! He was not a magistrate nor was he a judge. It was not for him to decide whether to take action or just caution a speeding motorist. His job was just to book a speeding motorist and leave his elders and betters to decide what action to take.

PC Jarvis and the other policeman had known of the dressing-down he had received, and when they realized another doctor had been trapped in the sergeant's net they had expected anything except a merciful outcome.

Time had healed the wound a little. Two weeks had elapsed since the dressing-down and being PC Jarvis's doctor had softened his resolve to mete out the death penalty.

I had evidently been a very lucky doctor that day.

By coincidence, I had another interesting experience in 1966 while driving along Nunhead Lane. It was six months after my brush with the police, this time I was driving in the opposite direction from Peckham Rye towards Consort Road.

I had just negotiated the bend in the road opposite Barforth Road, just a few yards from where on the opposite side of the road I had previously been caught in a speed trap, when I saw an elderly man sitting halfway up the wall at the corner of Consort Road and Nunhead Lane. This wall which has long since disappeared with the redevelopment of the area must originally have been seven feet high, but the top half had been demolished, and an old man was perched about five feet above the ground on the ragged bottom section. A load of bricks scattered indiscriminately all over the pavement under the wall showed that an accident had just happened.

I just could not believe my eyes! There appeared to be no other traffic in the àrea, no cars, no other person in sight, no noise, just a little old man sitting on top of a half knocked down wall. To describe him as sitting is not quite correct, he was more bent double than sitting and as he was facing the road he kept moving his head from side to side, as if he was trying to see something.

I stopped and got out of my car before I reached the spot. It was eerie, everything appeared unreal, it reminded me of a film set, but there were no lights or cameras to be seen. It was then that I saw and heard a lorry backing into Linden Grove, from Nunhead Lane. It had, as I later learned, hit this man, knocked the top of the wall down, and left him suspended on the unbroken part. The wall must have been in a pretty bad state for it to have disintegrated on impact which was fortunate for the little old man because otherwise he most certainly would have been crushed to death.

I helped the old chap down from the wall, and brushed him down as best I could for he was covered in dust. He was shaken and shocked, but who would not be having just had an argument with a ten ton lorry? From his appearance he looked as if he could do with a hospital check up, but he was still articulate and insisted that he was all right. Would I please take him home? However hard I tried to persuade him, he adamantly refused to go to hospital. It was then I had to be stubborn myself and make it a condition that if I took him home first to tell his wife that he was all right and not to worry, he would allow me to take him to hospital. He agreed. I took him home. In spite of the pleadings from both his wife and himself that they thought it unnecessary I insisted that he went to hospital. To make sure that he actually did as he was told, I took him to Dulwich Hospital casualty department myself. I explained to the casualty officer what I had seen, left him to notify the police, and decide himself after he had examined the chap whether the fellow required admission.

I then drove back along Nunhead Lane to do the home visits which had brought me along this route in the first place, when on reaching the spot where the accident had occurred I found a large crowd had gathered. There were two police cars, an ambulance, recovery van, fire engine, and also the lorry which had been the cause of all the trouble, in the immediate vicinity. All the occupants of these vehicles were looking for an injured man, who had been spirited away by an unknown force!

The lorry driver had reported the accident to the police, and given his version of the accident. His brakes had failed as he had approached the corner of Linden Grove and Nunhead Lane, and knew, now only thought he knew, he had knocked a man down. He just could not explain what had happened to the victim. He was almost certain he had hit someone, for he had tried to avoid the fellow, and in doing so had skidded and crashed into the wall. He believed he had done the right thing by calling an ambulance, but was now not so sure; there did not appear to be a victim. If there was one, he had not been seriously injured for he had got up and walked away.

When his lorry had come to a stop there had been a body on the wall; he was sure of it, he had backed his lorry into Linden Grove to rescue him. When he finally got down from his lorry the chap had gone. He thought the fellow must have fallen backwards on to the other side of the wall and had gone to help him, but couldn't find him. The chap had simply vanished into thin air. He was beginning to think the accident had affected his mental balance! I suppose he was hoping it was all a bad dream and that he would soon wake up.

I stopped, explained the situation to the police, and told them that I was the unknown force who had spirited the victim away and where he could now be found. The police thanked me for my prompt assistance to the victim and asked in the usual way to give my name and address. In hindsight, having done my bit of first aid, I should never have returned to the scene.

The victim was not a patient of mine, but out of interest I telephoned the hospital a fews days later to find out what the casualty officer had done and what injuries the victim had sustained. I learned he had been examined from head to foot, X-rayed, but having no bones broken, he had been discharged with a letter to the care of his own GP. The fellow had only suffered bruising, and as he denied he had ever lost consciousness, the casualty officer had no alternative but to accede to his wishes and allow the man to return to his home. As with all matters which were not my concern, I forgot all about the incident and it went completely out of my mind. I was very busy in the practice and this was just one incident in a busy daily work schedule.

Out of the blue, in 1969, three years after the affair of the broken wall, a firm of solicitors wrote to me asking for a report on the injuries sustained by their client who was now making a claim against the lorry driver. I had only made a superficial examination of the victim at the actual time of the accident and my report was consequently only a short one. The solicitors were not satisfied with my findings; they wrote to me again questioning my statement, they were obviously trying to get me to write that I had found their client half dead. I replied, but received no further communication from them until nine months later I was subpoenaed by them to appear in court as a witness.

Barristers are actors and can make or break a witness. They have it in their power if they are good and have the expertise to make one look so foolish as to make one want to run away and hide. I will never forget that court case. I had a horrible time. Even writing about it now a quarter of a century later evokes painful memories.

The barrister representing the old man resented my evidence that his client was conscious when I took him off the rubble. He was attempting to throw doubts on my remembrance of events which had taken place three years previously. At the time it seemed to me that I was being accused of giving false evidence.

'Surely doctor, you don't expect us to believe, this frail, old, man, you see him sitting here,' he then pointed to the old man, who seemed to have aged twenty years in the three years since I had last seen him, 'was fully in charge of his faculties, having suffered such a serious accident.'

He paused after every short statement: his speech was staccato: like sharp rapier thrusts. I was the victim! I winced.

'The wall was knocked down, doctor! It was a solid brick seven foot wall which had withstood the Blitz, doctor!'

Here he made a very lengthy pause, looked at the judge, then at me.

'The lorry was a ten tonner which had skidded! The man was in the middle of the road!'

I winced again. I was sweating. I had done nothing, why did I feel as if I was on trial?

He continued. 'This lorry, travelling at speed, had seen this poor old man and tried to stop. The driver found that his brakes had failed. He did all he could, but the lorry skidded. He then knocked this poor old man through the wall! Knocked the top of the wall down, doctor! He was suspended on top of it! You still insist that he was conscious and able to speak to you?'

The barrister was using short sharp sentences to give maximum effect to his oratory. It was obvious that he was doing his best to cast doubt on my evidence and at the time, I was, in the barrister's opinion, either lying, being paid by the defendants, or mentally defective for sticking to my evidence. I could only tell the truth, and as I continued to stick to my own version of what I had seen and done, the hostility shown to me by the barrister was almost more than I could bear.

The barrister was doing his best to break me, and he was succeeding. I was being ground into fine powder in a mill. My mind was in a whirl: as I continued to answer his questions, I reverted to the stammer from which I had suffered as a boy. I was not used to being in court and when I had been, I had certainly not been treated as a hostile witness. Whenever I had previously made a court appearance I had always been treated with deference, respect and friendliness; now I was being attacked. The judge too was allowing my persecution to continue without interference.

The barrister was after all only doing his duty. He was not medically qualified, and an old man perched on top of a broken down wall, placed there by a ten ton lorry, must have given him a field day for his acting abilities. I don't suppose for one moment he personally bore me any malice. In court however, from the way he kept looking at me, you would have thought he even resented the air that I breathed.

When I was allowed to leave the witness stand after giving my evidence and told that my presence in the court would no longer be required, I fled. To this day I do not know how the case ended, or how much the old man got in compensation. My mind was in a turmoil. I just wanted to forget that I had ever been involved. I had only stopped to help a poor chap who had been knocked down and was stuck on top of a wall. This was my reward for my good deed.

I did not even stop to collect my fee for my court appearance!

Hospitals in the fifties had a chain of command, with a matron, deputy matron and nurses – slaves. The slaves walked in awe when approached by their superiors, shuddered when they passed, and trembled at their commands. The matron was usually such a commanding figure that even the consultants treated her as if she was some tin-pot dictator.

On visiting the Oldfield family living in Lyndhurst Way in 1961, I was asked by a shrieking lady under the dining-room table to discuss the treatment I was giving to Mr Oldfield who had suffered a heart attack. At that time, heart attacks were generally treated at home with several weeks of bed rest followed by several weeks of recuperation. No one ever returned to work under three months.

The shrieking lady was seeking refuge from the three years old Oldfield boy who was attacking her with his little fists while she was attempting to evade his punches. Needless to say, I was very flippant in my answers to this lady. I simply did not believe Mrs Oldfield when she told me that this cowering being was the deputy matron of Dulwich Hospital.

I had a hernia operation in Dulwich Hospital in 1963 and my side ward was being especially spring-cleaned one morning: the 'goddess' was coming to visit me. It was not unusual for the matron to visit a GP in a hospital bed, and when she and her retinue duly appeared, we passed the time of day quite pleasantly.

On the following day, the spring-clean was repeated. When I asked why, I was informed that I was to be honoured by a visit on this occasion by the deputy matron. To my delight, the lady under the table in the Oldfield house reappeared, now dressed in her deputy matron's uniform, also followed by a retinue.

'You see,' she said laughing, 'I really do have a responsible position. The boy who was chasing me is my nephew. Mrs Oldfield is my sister.'

Thank heavens Mr Oldfield recovered. It would have done my reputation no good at all if he had succumbed.

The hernia operation in itself was nothing to write home about, except I remember being given the 'pre-med' in the anaesthetic room and becoming very sleepy. I was wheeled from the anaesthetic room into the operating theatre, and while on the operating table was asked by Mr Herriot, the surgeon, on which side the hernia was!

He must have been playing games with me. Although I found him to be a most charming man, he always wore the same serious expression. On waking up after the operation I examined my groins very carefully, to make sure that he had operated on the correct side. He had!

☆ ☆ ☆

On my visits to patients dogs have sometimes been friendly, sometimes too friendly, but they quickly realized that I was not there to play, nor did I fear them. After the initial bark they tended to ignore me.

On a home visit in February 1962 to Mr Blackmore, in Brayards Road, my lack of fear of dogs paid off. The Blackmores had been patients of mine from my first day in practice, but in ten years, if they had required attention they had come to the surgery. I had never crossed their doorstep as a doctor, only as a customer, to buy sweets for my children. They owned a sweet shop in which Mr Blackmore, his wife, or occasionally in the evening, his son served. The shop remained open until late in the evening, so on this February evening at 9 p.m., the shop was still open.

It was dark, cold, and miserable outside, and the shop was dimly lit. I went into the shop, the bell over the door clanged, the Blackmores knew they had a customer, but no one appeared behind the counter. I waited and waited, but no one answered my call; I opened the flap on the counter and slipped behind it.

I opened the glass dividing door between the shop and the living accommodation, to be met by a huge Alsatian, snarling, baring his teeth, yet slowly backing away. I pretended not to show any concern, and as I took one apprehensive step forward, this ferocious looking animal took one step backwards. It growled, snarled and barked the whole time. It never took its eyes off me. Needless to say, apart from the snarling and growling, I was behaving in the same fashion. I never took my eyes off the beast for one second. I held my medical bag in front of me in case the animal decided to change its conduct and make a dash forwards, instead of slowly retreating.

Mr Blackmore was lying on a couch at the end of the room, and the Alsatian, still snarling and baring its teeth, finally settled underneath him. To say that at this moment I was apprehensive at approaching a sick man's bed, would be an understatement.

Mr Blackmore, quite ill, had apparently been dozing while the dog and I had played out our scene, but with the snarling immediately underneath him, suddenly woke up and saw me. He apologized for not being able to open the door, and for his wife not being in. She had just popped out to a neighbour, and I had come rather sooner than she had thought. He was in a pool of sweat: I was in a sweat too, wondering which part of my anatomy his dog would attack first when I came to examine his master.

He had given no orders to the dog, and I had to pretend to be brave, that there was nothing amiss. I examined him, while the dog continued a low pitched growl under the couch.

'Normally he would have bitten you,' Mr Blackmore suddenly said, as I had my stethoscope on his chest listening to his heart, and my eyes fixed firmly on the dog under the couch. I was shocked.

'Why didn't you tell me you had a dangerous animal?' I asked.

'No problem,' he answered. 'He would only have been dangerous if you had come last week. Today he is scared of you. You remind him of the vet who came a couple of days ago. He had a bag like yours, when the dog saw you he thought you were the vet. We called the vet because the dog had an abscess in his mouth, and when the vet came, the dog went for him. The vet however must be used to this behaviour. He is a big muscular man; he grabbed hold of Rod's head under his arm, saw the cause of the abscess, a bad tooth in his mouth, and yanked it out! He has backed away from you, he doesn't want to lose another tooth.'

In 1964 I was working with a partner, Dr Kwasny, who had such a friendly personality he attracted patients to him. He was such a nice chap that I was not surprised one evening to hear this deaf old lady, Mrs Law, shouting to the receptionists that she wanted to see him. She definitely did not want to see me.

I knew her well, she was in her eighties, and I had been a regular visitor to her home for years. I recognized her voice immediately as it reverberated through the surgery premises. She was as deaf as a doorpost, a cantankerous old dear, who lived with her husband in the Palyns Alms Houses in Choumert Road. This evening, she definitely did not want to see me. I distinctly heard her say so!

'I don't want to see that bleeder Dr Crown, he's bloody useless.'

The receptionist was arguing with her, but besides being deaf Mrs Law refused to listen. I distinctly heard the receptionist say that Dr Kwasny was not on duty, that it was his half day, and that I was the only doctor available. Both parties were rapidly losing patience when Mrs Law suddenly shouted that although she was dissatisfied, hated me, there was no choice, and in the circumstances, as she required urgent attention, she would see me.

I had heard this commotion, no one on the premises had failed to hear it and the patients in the waiting room were killing themselves with laughter. I was however to be the victim of her hatred, and it would be an understatement to remark that I was not terribly thrilled at having to see her. I wondered what fate was awaiting me.

I ushered her in to my room when her turn came with a large smile, pretending that I had heard nothing. She greeted me with the words, 'I hate you I do! Do you want to know why? You keep my old bugger alive you do.'

I then understood why she hated me. Her poor old aged husband had eight weeks previously had a heart attack. I had managed to save him!

☆ ☆ ☆

The surgery is situated in an area where violence, unknown in my early years, has become in the past twenty years a way of life. We count ourselves lucky that we are in the better part of Peckham, on the East Dulwich border, and have not suffered quite as much as other areas.

Many of our patients live in more disturbed zones where violence is a daily occurrence; in Bellenden Road itself I can only remember five armed raids!

One, in the sub-post office opposite the surgery, in the 1970s, the postmaster was bundled into a van, but not before the raiders had shut his right hand in the van door. He was severely beaten up in this raid before he agreed to hand over the keys, and the injury he suffered to his hand resulted in the loss of all the fingers. This attack had such a severe effect on him that he never returned to work, the post office was closed, and he died of a heart attack a year or so later.

The sweet shop at 119 Bellenden Road was raided by an armed gangster in 1984, when the terrified shopkeeper was 'requested' to hand over the till money. A man walking past the shop saw what was happening inside through the shop window, and with remarkable bravery managed to close and make fast the shop door, to trap the raider inside. He hoped by doing this to buy enough time for the police to arrive. The gangster, realizing that it would be pointless to attempt to escape by the now closed door grabbed the till money and propelled himself through the plate glass window. He arrived on the pavement outside still holding his gun: he made good his escape, but left a bloody trail.

Our local jeweller, at 125 Bellenden Road, Mr Nash, affectionately known as 'Dee', was held at gun point about fifteen years ago, but only a small amount of jewellery was stolen. Clocks and watches of little value were taken as he did not have the keys of the safe full of jewellery on him. The safe was so heavy that the armed raiders however hard they tried just could not move it. They had evidently made arrangements for its removal unopened; they had brought a special van with them. Perhaps he would have been more fortunate if he had held the keys and they had taken the jewellery. They were so angry and frustrated with him, they split his head open with a sawn off shot-gun. He never recovered from this traumatic experience, he abandoned his shop, moved out of the area, and I have heard recently that he has died.

Iris, a Jamaican lady, who owned the fruit shop a few doors away from the surgery was held up at gunpoint by an armed gang in 1970. They demanded the till money, but instinctively, instead of giving it to them, she screamed for help. Her husband, who was upstairs in their flat over the shop at the time promptly answered her call. He stood at the top of the stairs, out of sight, shouted down to the raiders to take the money and not to hurt his wife. He had no intention of coming to her rescue, perhaps he was wise not to do so, but she has never forgiven him. They are now divorced. To be fair, Iris and her husband had been at daggers drawn over his involvement with a member of the fair sex before this incident, the attack was just another contributory factor in their breakup.

It was a cold November night in 1982 and I was in my consulting room examining a patient when I heard dogs barking. My consulting room is situated in a purpose-built chalet in the garden of 105 Bellenden Road, the barking dogs sounded as if they were outside my back door. On opening the door, I saw policemen with torches, and dogs on leads, in the next door garden, two yards away from me. This house was empty at the time and the policemen looked suspiciously at me until they saw the stethoscope round my neck. They then explained they were looking for an armed raider who had eluded them after a hold-up in the area. They knew that he was trying to make his escape through the gardens, and wondered whether I had seen or heard him. I searched the garden shed with them: they found no intruder, and I returned to continue with my consultations as though the episode was a normal pattern of life.

I must admit, I felt very sorry for the police. They were unarmed, looking for an armed man! They looked pale and apprehensive; who wouldn't when faced with an armed fugitive on the run? They sent their dogs into the neighbouring gardens, and eventually he was caught in a garden shed six gardens away without anyone being hurt.

Patients and staff in the surgery had not been aware anything untoward had occurred.

It is a custom of many tribes to arrange their own funerals before they die. Tribal chiefs are always buried according to their traditional beliefs. One can arrange in some parts of America to have one's body deep-frozen, until scientists achieve the ultimate, and bring the body back to life. The Pyramids and the Taj Mahal are memorials of man's enterprise, in perpetuating the memory of the dead. The Cave of Machpelloh in Hebron, bought for four hundred shekels by Abraham from Ephrom the Hittite is a story I have always remembered. It was a freehold purchase in the state of Israel.

Burials and memorials are never far from a doctor's life, but what did surprise me was when Mrs Lawrence told me in 1988 that she had booked her own funeral and wanted my approval. As she was sixty-eight years old at the time, and not seriously ill, I wondered whether she was telling me something I did not know. Perhaps she had been to a clairvoyant who had informed her what a lousy doctor I was, and hinted at a diagnosis which I had missed. I made no remark, just grinned as she carried on; the cost was going to be eight hundred pounds, she said.

It was going to be the funeral of her dreams! She had chosen the coffin, cream wood, varnished, lined in lemon padded silk. Did I know, she remarked, that some undertakers use materials that are rough on the skin. I smiled a sickly grin and asked why the padding. She anwered without blinking. 'I took the undertaker's advice, he said thick padding would save me a bumpy ride!'

Coffins, she explained, came in all sizes and shapes. She had heard of one body which had been too long for the coffin and had been doubled up to fit. A coffin had to be wide enough too, if one wanted space enough to breathe. There was nothing worse than being in an uncomfortable coffin, lying there to eternity. I listened to her spellbound; she meant every word she said; there was not a hint of facetiousness in her remarks.

The undertaker was an excellent salesman; he deserved every bit of credit for his powers of persuasion. He told her that the price for the 'performance' was a bargain. It was a set price, and included VAT: with rising inflation she had made an excellent investment. There was one snag: the funeral directors had made the transaction non-transferable; it was exclusive to her body. No one else could use the receipt. Should she die in Guatemala, for example, she would lose her money. She had to die in the United Kingdom. Since the burial was to take place in Honor Oak Crematorium, the undertakers had agreed to bring her body back from anywhere outside London, at no extra cost!

I made no comment. Not only had the salesman been able to persuade her to buy a superior coffin, he had had the *chutzpah* to make her believe she was to lie in her coffin to eternity – after having been cremated!

She had paid cash down. She would be allowed two cars plus a hearse for the price. To make sure she had the perfect funeral she had taken the precaution of giving her son a sum of money for extra cars. She had many friends and was sure that the money would be needed. Most of her friends were old and did not have cars of their own. She had given her son the receipt from the undertakers. All was now ready for the great send-off. She actually said she was looking forward to it.

Perhaps I am morbid, but her enthusiasm rather

escaped me!

☆ ☆ ☆

Holly Grove crosses Bellenden Road, at one end of the Grove is Rye Lane, which is the main shopping centre in Peckham; at the other end is Warwick Gardens, which was, before it was renamed, part of Azenby Road. Holly Grove also houses the Shrubbery and several houses of character which time has not changed.

Facing the Shrubbery, the house with a wooden entrance door to the basement covered with iron on its backside intrigued me the most. It was number 22, owned by Mrs John. The iron-clad door had presumably been made in this fashion when the house was built, to prevent highwaymen who might have tried to hack the door down from the outside.

The house had been built in 1840; Mr John had bought it in 1913, but I never knew this gentleman; he had departed this life long before my arrival in Peckham. Mrs John lived on the ground floor of this house: she was a shrivelled up miserly old lady, in her eighties, who would only buy sixpennyworth of chips from the local fish and chip shop, although everyone in the area knew that she was a very wealthy woman. It was common knowledge that old Mr John had left his missus well provided for!

The sixpennyworth of chips bought on Monday was made to last her for the whole week. She boiled six eggs on Monday, to save money on the gas bill; she then had six suppers for the week. Her diet never varied: one pennyworth of chips and one egg for supper every weekday. Sunday was the Lord's day so she splashed out a little and allowed herself a lamb chop.

When in 1954 she took ill and I prescribed a greater

variety to her diet, she told me this was impossible; she was saving her money. The greatest thrill in her life she told me would be, if after she was dead, she was able to leave a larger inheritance to her grandson than the other grandparents. Her logic defeated me; how would she know after she was dead?

She rented the basement of her house to the Runacres, and although Mrs Runacre has now died and most of her family no longer live in the area I still maintain contact; one of the sons is still a patient of mine and I see him regularly. There was no love lost between the Runacres and Mrs John. As I have already pointed out she was a miserly old skin-flint, only interested in saving money, and spent all her waking hours in working out ways of doing so. This meant persecuting the Runcares, they were her tenants and made to know it and had to be kept in their place. The Runacres attributed her miserliness to eccentricity, due to age, and would run errands for the old lady as an act of kindness. She was after all in her eighties; the Runacres, not knowing the contents of her will, genuinely felt sorry for her.

The Runacres moved into the basement of No. 22 in 1945, but Mr Runacre died in 1956, and his wife afterwards had to cope with the situation as best she could. Mrs Runacre was in her fifties when her husband died, and she was in the unenviable position of not being able to afford to move and having living accommodation most unsuitable for her growing family. This basement was dark, miserable and damp. The Runacres had attempted for years to get Mrs John to rent them one of her empty rooms on an upstairs floor, without success: on this occasion her malevolence was greater than her miserliness.

Mrs Runacre had no option to stick it out until Mrs John died in 1960 when she took the law into her own hands and moved from the damp basement upstairs. There then proceeded a long court case over possession with the heir to the property in which I became involved as Mrs Runacre's doctor. Mrs Runacre won in the end. The court findings only gave her the right to retain the upstairs while she herself remained in the building; her family were given no rights; it could be said therefore that both parties were victorious.

Mrs Runacre however lived until 1981 so had many years living in a dry environment. When she died, Mrs John's dreams were fulfilled; her heir took over the whole of the house. Mrs John can indeed rest in peaceful bliss; she fulfilled her dream; she had managed to leave her grandson more than his other grandparents had.

Facing the side of the road in which the Runcares lived is the Shrubbery, which as its name implies, is a small park filled with shrubs. When the Johns bought their house this Shrubbery was a private park owned by the tenants of Holly Grove which was kept locked. Each householder in the Grove had a key; the common herd were kept out! The Shrubbery is now a public park, a home for birds, swings for the children, a place for my patients to sit in the summer, and a meeting and sleeping place for the meths and cider drinkers of the area. The memory of the past however still refuses to leave, its railing and gates remain, and it is still kept locked at night.

Next door to the Runacres lived Mr and Mrs Moorgate who joined my National Health list in 1962. They were a couple in their late forties who had worked for the colonial service, and had just returned from a period of residence in the backwoods of South America.

In June of that year I had an occasion to visit Mr Moorgate. I went upstairs to his bedroom and, knowing the previous residences of the Moorgates, I was not surprised to find various totem poles, drums and other nicknacks of his tours on my way up. What did surprise me, shocked is the correct word, was to find a wooden coffin underneath the window bay of his bedroom. Lying in bed, he could dream of his future!

I looked at the patient, looked at his wife, looked at the coffin again, and with a grin said to Mrs Moorgate, 'It's pointless examining your old man or giving you a prescription, you've got everything stitched up. If you hang on I will go to the surgery and bring back a death certificate with me. It will hasten his departure.'

I knew the couple well, knew they had a sense of humour similar to mine, otherwise, I would have been in serious trouble for making such facetious remarks.

The coffin I was told was not a fake; it was a real one, made of sandalwood with wooden handles. It was now being used by the Moorgates as a chest for storing linen, but it had not been bought originally for this purpose.

The history of this chest (coffin) was that Mr Moorgate had contracted sandfly fever whilst working in the civil service in one of the remote villages in the mountains of South America. What a British civil servant should be doing working in such a remote place I never asked, and as they did not volunteer the information I thought it prudent not to question. He had been there for two years when he was struck down: people in the area died so quickly of sandfly fever it was natural for a coffin to be made for the sufferer as soon as he had contracted the disease. Most of the sufferers made use of theirs, but Mr Moorgate was a tough bloody-minded Englishman who, according to the locals, did not have the decency to fill his. One had been made for him, but he was one of the survivors. Rather than waste a good wooden container he had brought it home with him and used it as a chest for storing linen. He had brought it over with him from South America using it as a cabin trunk; the baggage labels were still affixed to its sides.

He said he had no intention of throwing it out. It had cost him good money, one day he was going to save money by using it for its proper purpose. Thankfully, I was saved the prospect of having to argue the matter out with him; the Moorgates moved in 1978, and I have never heard from them since.

I don't believe I would have had the courage to sleep in the same room as my ultimate resting place, however much money I was going to save.

☆ ☆ ☆

Mrs Flowers owned a flower shop in Peckham Rye and became a private patient of mine in the 1970s. For me, at that time, to have a regular private patient was like finding a pot of gold. She was a descendant of a long line of flower sellers as her family had been in the flower trade for generations. As they had lived in the area too, her business was a well-known and well-established one. Her main work was making wreaths, sheaves and wedding bouquets, and I would watch her with her nimble fingers weaving greenery and flowers in wire frames. She would keep talking to me at the same time as describing her symptoms, so as not to waste time and concentration. The end result of her work showed that her concentration had not been affected by my visits. Incidentally, this establishment, long since closed down, made my daughter's wedding bouquet, also provided flowers for the *chupah* in the South-East London District Synagogue.

At my daughter's wedding, Mr Michael O'Shea, a patient, a devout Catholic, who played the organ in the local Catholic church was persuaded by me to play the organ in the synagogue. I believe I pacified his conscience and overcame his reluctance by informing him that Dr and Mrs Healy, well-known to him as devout co-religionists, would also be at the ceremony. He was sufficiently reassured by their presence that he would not be rewarded with eternal damnation for his synagogue appearance!

I first became acquainted with Mrs Flowers when she was already over seventy years of age and she had already been ill for some years. She was dissatisfied with her previous doctor's treatment and her niece, who had been a National Health patient of mine for some years, had recommended me to her. The difficulty was that the old lady just could not spare the time and had not the patience to be ill, and I had great problems in persuading her to take part in any investigations. She only finally agreed to be seen by a hospital consultant with the greatest reluctance, and investigations proved her to be much more seriously ill than either of us had thought. She required to be given a weekly injection and this for me at the time proved to be not such a hardship: the most suitable day for her was Friday which meant my wife had a bunch of flowers to grace our home every weekend.

She was a very generous lady. I remember her giving me an envelope in 1972, the day before I was going on holiday, making me promise not to open it until I was airborne. I was going to Israel with the family at the time, but to say that I purposely respected her wishes would not be truthful. I put the envelope in my inside jacket pocket expecting it to contain a happy holiday message, and promptly forgot all about it. I did not remember it until I was sitting relaxed in the aeroplane. When I opened the envelope I found to my astonishment that inside the card wishing me a happy holiday was tucked one hundred pounds, in five pound notes. In 1972 each person was only allowed to take out of the country fifty pounds as a travel allowance and I already had the maximum amount with me. What my explanation would have sounded like to the customs officials if they had decided to search me, I dread to think. They certainly would not have believed the truth.

As Mrs Flowers's condition slowly deteriorated she demanded more and more of my time and attention. My visits to her were increased to twice weekly, and in the final period to three times weekly. She still however struggled on in her business although now she was no longer capable of doing the manual work. The making of wreaths and wedding bouquets she left to her niece, Daphne, while she kept the accounts.

Besides work, Mrs Flowers had one other pleasure in life - cigarettes - she chain-smoked. At the time I was smoking a pipe myself, and I was therefore not able to pressurize her as much as I should have done to discontinue this habit. In any event her illness was in no way related to smoking or her chest, and I was forced to be a bystander and watch as one cigarette followed another. Her fingers were stained, not from the flowers which she wove into her wreaths, but from the nicotine-staining of the cigarettes which never left her fingers.

One Saturday, in 1976, the telphone rang at eight o'clock in the morning in my house. This was an extremely rare occurrence. I always took Saturday morning as my half day, and the housekeeper at the surgery had strict instructions not to disturb me. There was always another doctor on duty. When my wife who had answered the telephone asked me to speak to the caller, I knew there had to be something seriously wrong.

It was Daphne's husband, Albert, who requested an

urgent visit to Mrs Flowers. He had been telephoned by a friend of his who lived in Copeland Road, just yards away from the Flowers' flower shop, that the flower shop was on fire and fire engines were there. I knew Albert lived out of the area and did not drive a car so I could not refuse him when he asked me as a favour to find out what had happened to his aunty. It would be much quicker for me to get to her he said than to wait until he could make his way to Peckham. I went immediately, but by the time I arrived at the shop the fire brigade was ready to leave and the salvage vehicle had arrived.

The shop was flooded, and there was an overpowering smell of charred and burned wood. The only occupant was a policeman poking about the charred wood where the counter had previously stood. I quickly learned from him that it was believed the old lady had smoked in bed and had accidentally set fire to the place. It was presumed that in her attempts to escape from a fire in her bedroom she had fallen down the stairs: she had been found burnt to death on the first floor landing.

Mrs Flowers's living accommodation on the two floors over the shop had been large and luxurious. Her dining-room, lounge and kitchen, all extremely well-furnished, had been on the first floor. Her bedroom on the second floor had a characteristic which I had never previously seen, and which I have never seen since. In the inside folds of the heavy velvet curtains which covered her windows were pinned envelopes; inside these envelopes were five and ten pound notes.

I found out the envelope phenomenon quite accidentally. One evening she sent for me to give her something to ease her abdominal pain and I had no alternative but to give her an injection of morphine. She was in bed, she would after the injection shortly be asleep, and I suggested to her that I draw the curtains. It was then that I noticed the 'hangings'. She noticed my amazement, and her excuse for hiding the money in this fashion was that she did not trust her bank manager with her money.

Mrs Flowers had already been removed to the mortuary in the Borough and I was asked by the police to go and identify her. No relative or anyone who knew her had as yet appeared. The police said, as I had known her so well that it would spare the relatives from a sight they would never forget. They were right!

I went to the mortuary and it was a most distressing experience to see a lady whom I had known and admired, 'roasted'. Roasted or toasted are the only descriptions I can offer which met my gaze that morning.

Returning home from the mortuary, as my children had not yet returned from the synagogue and it was too late to join them, I said my sabbath prayers at home with the smell of burning flesh and charred wood in my nostrils. When my children came home my wife served up for the family sabbath dinner cold roast chicken, the skin of which had been nicely browned.

I ran from the room! I felt violently sick! I skipped that meal. Even today, when I am confronted with cold roast chicken, my memory floods back to that year of 1976.

In 1989, when Hannah Chesney told me the story of her bizarre upbringing she had, in spite of it, reached the mature age of ninety-six years.

Apart from the natural wear and tear which follows the ageing process her memory of times and events was faultless and she enjoyed having political discussions with me. She had arthritis, but was still able to get about and do her own housework. The only external help she needed apart from the occasional visit from me was with her shopping. She had all her faculties and I always enjoyed visiting her, even though at times she was blunt to the point of rudeness.

After my mother's death in 1986 I followed the orthodox Jewish custom of not shaving for the first thirty days after the funeral. I had not reckoned on being asked to visit Hannah with a twenty-five day growth of hair on my face. She answered the door, and stared at my stubbly face in disbelief. She did not bother to greet me with her usual smile, just pointed to my face and blurted out, 'What the hell do you think you're playing at? That can bloody well come off!'

After I had explained the reason for my unkempt facial appearance she was full of remorse, did her best to comfort me at my loss, and apologized for her lack of knowledge of Jewish customs.

Hannah was born in 1894, in Westmoreland Road, Walworth, and her father was known in the area as 'Handsome Jack' the lady-killer. He moved the family to Grosvenor Terrace, Camberwell in 1900, when she was six years old, and as her childhood consisted of constant changes of address she became a child of the streets. Hannah it can be said had a true Dickensian upbringing.

She never had a proper home. The furniture in her home consisted of orange boxes, and the family slept on old mattresses on the floor. Crockery did not exist in her parents' home. They used condensed milk tins as cups. They would buy a tin of condensed milk for a halfpenny, take off the lid, then file down the rough edges, to prevent their lips being cut. Her father rarely paid the rent, and the family more often than not would find themselves homeless – thrown out into the street.

Her father was a violent man who physically abused her mother, and her mother was so severely beaten up by him on one occasion that her jaw was fractured and she had to be hospitalized. He would come home drunk, or from a night out with a girl friend, then demand food. When there was none available he would ask for money: when both requests were refused her mother would receive a good beating. He would often steal from her mother the means to entertain his many lady friends, and Hannah's hatred of her father began at an age when most girls have an affection for Dad.

When her mother was in hospital with a fractured jaw, her father came home one day, left Hannah to care for herself, and took Hannah's brother and younger sister away with him. She never saw her father again, neither did she see her sister until after Hannah herself was married.

Hannah, with her mother in hospital, now left on her own, slept in the street at the entrance of their old home. Her grandmother came to visit one day not knowing of the family breakup and finding Hannah in her sorry state took her to live with her. She lived with her grandmother until she was twenty-one years old then went into service as a housekeeper to an army officer's family.

She learned some years later that her father in a fit of temper had killed her brother with a poker and had been sentenced to a long term of imprisonment. She now cannot remember what the exact sentence was, and she also does not know what happened to him after he served his prison sentence. I was rather distressed to hear her say that she hoped his end had been a bad one.

It is really rather sad that an old lady of such a great age should still feel so bitter and bear such hatred towards one of her parents. In normal circumstances time or death is usually the healer of such deep wounds.

9

Spanish Holiday

Some people never seem to have any luck; misfortune always appears to be their lot.

In the 1960s, we frequently had outbreaks of smallpox, and governments took precautions against importing this killer disease. If you went abroad most countries required an incoming traveller to provide a valid certificate of vaccination against smallpox. Sometimes the foreign country was not so concerned as we were and in order to return you had to provide one: we did not want to import the disease.

When a smallpox epidemic broke out anywhere in the world the recommendation of the Ministry of Health to doctors in this country was to vaccinate as many people as possible. I spent many Sundays vaccinating patients who had no intention or the means of leaving Peckham, never mind leaving this country.

In 1968, Alan, a bachelor, twenty-seven years old, booked a holiday in Spain, and came to see me about smallpox vaccination. He however made it plain that he had no intention of paying for an international certificate; it was his right as a National Health patient to receive one for nothing. Incidentally, at the time I only charged half-a-crown for one. He refused to have his vaccination done, he thought he was being overcharged, and we did not part on the best of terms. He told me that doctors were wealthy enough, he had never met a poor one, and he had no intention of making this one any wealthier. I had always known Alan for his quick temper, and he left me in a fury to go to one of the immunization centres of British European Airways. He refused to be done there too, he was beside himself with rage when they told him that their charge was a guinea! He told me so himself, many months later, after we had patched up our friendship. He therefore went to Spain without being vaccinated.

On his arrival in Spain late at night he was asked to show his international certificate. Not being able to produce one he was locked up in the airport prison overnight. The reason for this incarceration was that there was no doctor available at that time of night to vaccinate him. It was hot, stuffy and smelly in that most inhospitable enclosure – he spent a most uncomfortable night.

In the morning a doctor arrived, and he was told that if he wished to enter the country he had to be vaccinated there and then. The charge would be the equivalent of twenty pounds. I have already mentioned that Alan was quick tempered; he now flew into a rage, had a bitter argument with the doctor over the extortionate amount he was being asked to pay, and again refused to be vaccinated.

'After all,' he said, when he later told me the story, 'twenty pounds is an enormous sum of money. I told the Spanish doctor I could have had it done in England for half-a-crown, and "the bastard" just laughed in my face.'

The doctor was accompanied by a policeman. They went out, not however before they had made sure the door was locked and bolted behind them. They left poor Alan to stew.

The policeman returned a few hours later with some horrible food, the sight of which made him want to vomit, and some drinking water which had become warm from standing in the heat. The policeman seemed friendly enough, but couldn't speak a word of English, and no amount of effort on Alan's part with sign language helped the situation. The policeman left the food, grinned from ear to ear as Alan was talking or making signs, locked the door behind him, and went away. Alan by this time was prepared to pay any amount of money to get out.

He was hot, sweaty, hungry and thirsty. He had not had a wash for two days. He was feeling so ghastly that when the doctor and the accompanying policeman returned at five o'clock that evening he agreed to be vaccinated!

The doctor, who spoke presentable English, now told him that beside the peseta equivalent of twenty pounds for the vaccination he would now have to pay for his board and lodging. This would cost another ten pounds: if he did not have enough currency, the doctor would be prepared to accept traveller's cheques. Alan had no choice. He would either have to remain incarcerated for goodness knows how long, with mounting charges for board and lodging, or pay ransom money. He paid the ransom, paid it in cash, was vaccinated, and continued his holiday.

The weather outside the prison cell was glorious, the sun shone, and there was not a cloud in the sky. It was lovely and warm in the fresh evening air. Even though he only had twenty pounds left out of his allowance of fifty pounds, his hotel accommodation, which included full board, had already been paid for in England. He would have to budget, but would only require the minimum for spending money, and would have to forget about buying any presents to take home.

Thirty pounds of his hard-earned allowance had gone to an avaricious Spanish doctor; he was now certain all doctors were tarred with the same brush. They were all crooked; he had seen the Spanish doctor share his money with the policeman; the police were no better. He was certain that he had been taken for a ride! He was in no position however to do anything about it and for once in his life became philosophical about his circumstances. He put his temper in his pocket, and went on to his hotel. There he met a German girl, and as he told me the story much later, he had a smashing time.

Alan, I have forgotten to mention, was an extremely good-looking young man; tall, six foot in height and athletic. He was also conceited enough to know that he would have no problem in finding a playmate at any holiday hotel which he would honour with his presence. This is why, in spite of his early problems, he had decided to continue his holiday. Indeed, he enjoyed his holiday in Spain so much, he decided to go again in the following year.

He intended to travel alone; he had been in correspondence with last year's flame and was going to spend his holiday with her again. This time however he was going to avoid buying trouble and he decided to go by car. His experience of Spanish doctors had been so illuminating that he now regarded me as an angel, and had made friends with me again. He even asked me to help him plan his journey and having been through France to Italy and Switzerland myself by car I was only too happy to help.

He made an overnight stop in France, in the hotel which I recommended, and arrived in Spain early next morning feeling fine, singing at the top of his voice. A few miles from the border he saw what appeared to him to be an injured man lying by the roadside. He stopped the car to help, but when he reached the man, who appeared to be elderly, the man started screaming in Spanish, pointing to Alan's car. Alan, who does not speak a word of Spanish – he does speak a few words of German learned from his German girlfriend, the girl he had met the previous year – could not understand what the man was shouting about. He kept looking at the man, then at his car, trying to decipher what the man was pointing at.

Within two minutes, a police squad car pulled up. A policeman got out, pointed to Alan and said, 'You German?'

'No!' said Alan, 'I'm English.'

The policeman took out his notebook and in broken English said, 'You travel fast, hit man where in road?'

Alan was stupefied. 'I didn't hit anyone,' he said.

The man, who had stopped his awful noise while listening intently to the conversation now started screaming again. He pointed to his leg, and the bumper of Alan's car. A second policeman, old, round, greasy and fat (Alan's venomous description), now slowly eased his bulk out of the squad car and started walking with slow intimidating steps round Alan's car. He was going through the motions of looking for damage, and was being helped in his search by the screaming man, who was pointing to a minute dent in Alan's bumper. The dent was just visible to the naked eye and had obviously been caused by a stone. But how could Alan explain this to policemen who were not prepared to listen to him, and pretended not to understand English? They looked at Alan when he spoke, as one may look at an idiot. Whenever he opened his mouth to speak, the policemen looked at each other, laughed, and ignored him.

'This very bad!' the second policeman said: this was referring to Alan's bumper.

Neither policeman seemed at all interested in the victim's injuries, or made any attempt to treat his fictitious wounds. In broken English the first policeman now told Alan that he would have to take him to the police station for questioning.

Poor Alan was in a cold sweat, hoping that any minute he would wake up from this terrible dream. He could not make any sense at all out of the situation. He did not know what was happening, where to turn for help; everything was so unreal. He was completely shattered!

Whilst Alan was in this numbed state the second policeman finally appeared to have found it his duty to go over to the 'injured' man. The policeman and the 'injured' man jabbered to each other in Spanish for five minutes; Alan just looked on, and sweated. The second policeman went over to the first and chatted to him, for what appeared to Alan to be hours. The first policeman suddenly appeared to break up the dialogue and came over to Alan to translate the contents of the conversation.

The poor injured man, whom Alan had nearly killed by his reckless driving, had a wife and four children to support. Alan was lucky; had he killed the man, he would now be on a murder charge. His minor injuries, no thanks to Alan, wholly due to the blessed saints, had not proved fatal. The injured fellow really did not want to spend his time in a police station; he felt so ill, he just wanted to return to his family as quickly as possible, and rest. The main injuries to his legs and spine would stop this poor man from working for three to four weeks. If Alan would give the poor injured chap, whom the saints in their mercy had preserved, the Spanish equivalent of forty pounds, four weeks' pay, he would drop any charges. He told Alan he was lucky he had knocked down such a saintly man, the injured chap was not even insisting on forcing Alan to pay for the cost of medical treatment.

Alan sized up the situation in a flash. The previous year's plane episode over vaccination sprung to his mind; he had been in a similar situation before. This time he did not hesitate, he gave the policeman forty pounds' worth of pesetas, did a U-turn, and belted out of Spain as fast as he could.

He telephoned the German girl whom he had arranged to meet in Spain as soon as he found himself able to do so, from a restaurant in France. This was ten hours after he should have arrived at the rendezvous, but she had not wasted any time. She had not waited for Alan; she had already found herself another beau in the hotel. He swore vengeance against Spain, the Spanish police and the Spanish people, vowing never to go back. He never has! He was also not feeling too happy about Germans, especially the frauleins.

Alan was a car salesman, a very good one, and a chap who earned a lot of money. However, instead of getting married he preferred to play the field. He lived with his widowed mother whom he adored; this may have been a factor as to why he never got married. When I once asked his mother why she did not go with Alan on holiday her reply was succinct, rapier-like, 'Leave England? Never!'

In the following year, in 1970, Alan to get away from his mother's apron strings for a couple of weeks, went abroad again. He kept his word, he did not go to Spain; he went to Portugal instead.

I saw him six weeks after his holiday in Portugal; he was looking very sorry for himself, feeling very stupid, and very low. He had gone in August, this was the only time his firm would give him a holiday, as it was a quiet time for car sales. He had known it was not the best time in the year to go to Portugal; it was going to be very hot, but he had no choice.

He arrived in Portugal early in the morning on the first day of his holiday after a very pleasant early morning flight, and went straight into this beautiful hotel overlooking the beach. He had breakfast, a few beers, put on his bathing costume and, having eaten and drunk a little too much, decided to lie down in a deckchair on the glorious warm sand in front of the hotel.

He went to sleep, and woke up in hospital later that day with a saline drip in his arm. The stupid idiot had not realized that it is dangerous to fall asleep in the hot sun without first becoming acclimatized. He had got so severely burnt that he had blistered. He had become so dehydrated that he had gone unconscious in his deckchair. He was told later by the hospital doctors that he was lucky to be alive, he had gone into renal failure.

Some hotel guests late that afternoon, frolicking about in front of the hotel, had accidentally knocked his deckchair down, and tipped poor Alan out. They were full of apologies, but Alan hadn't protested, just lay on the sand where he had fallen. They called an ambulance thinking that he had been severely injured in the fall, but although they were wrong in their diagnosis, they were instrumental in saving his life. He was rushed to hospital and was there for three weeks.

When I saw him he was still feeling weak and sickly; he had only come to see me for a sick certificate. He told me that the Portugal trip was the most expensive one he had ever had. It had cost him a lot of money, and he had been forced to borrow money from his friends to pay for the hospital expenses. Young and healthy as he was, he had not bothered to take out any medical insurance. As he explained to me, I knew he had never had a serious illness in his life and, as a physical fitness fanatic, had no intention of ever having one. The episode in Portugal had been exceptional; it had been due to tiredness, beer and sun.

I thought it unfair to ask him how Portugal compared with Spain, but at least in our conversation he did not blame the Portuguese for his costly adventure.

I asked where he was going on holiday the following year: he had obviously rehearsed the answer.

'Blackpool!'

He was going with Mom and playing safe.

I advised him to wear his heaviest clothing. Although he was going in August, knowing his luck he would come back with frost-bite. I do not think at that moment he appreciated my facetiousness; his smile was a forced one.

When I recall the series of misfortunes which befell him, if only he had agreed to pay 'this wealthy doctor' half-a-crown in the first instance for his vaccination, none of these crises would have occurred!

10

Booze and Bets

Mr Deveson, who was the owner of the Hope Public House in Rye Lane until he retired in the 1970s, was a character of the old school. He was the proprietor for thirty-two years, always wore a bow tie, was always immaculately dressed in the height of fashion, and was never lost for lady admirers.

When I first became acquainted with him it had not stretched my imagination to believe all the stories of his being a lady-killer. He was in his sixties, still a most handsome man with a charming personality. Before the Hope had come under his proprietorship he had lived with his parents in the Bun House in Peckham High Street which his father had owned since 1911.

The Bun House had some interesting traditions, which had been initiated in the 1920s and had continued until 1960. On Christmas Day, the carver from Simpsons in the Strand came especially to carve the turkey. It also had another tradition, on New Year's Day, when the poor of the community were given a free dinner, consisting of boiled beef, carrots, pease pudding and a piece of crusty bread. This New Year's Day dinner was served from 11 a.m.-3 p.m. All were welcome, no questions were asked. The area has never been short of poor people, and the walls of the Bun House on New Year's Day were bursting at the seams. The owner of the Bun House was well-known in the community for his charitable work, and his son, the chap I knew, when he became the owner of the Hope followed in his father's footsteps.

Whilst ninety-nine per cent of his customers did not even have the wherewithal to own an old jalopy Mr Deveson junior drove a Rolls Royce. His friends however were working-class Peckhamites, and such was his character, he did not have an ounce of pomposity in him. No one who entered his bar in need of a few shillings ever left empty-handed.

Many of my patients frequented his bar daily, in the morning, to place their bets with a bookie's runner. As horse or dog-race betting was illegal except at the race-track, or by telephone, the bookie's runner sat or stood in the public bar collecting bets. His trusted clients, surreptitiously slipped bits of paper into his hand with their bets and money which he took to the bookmaker. Winners were paid out in the bar on the following day, just as illegally!

Mr Deveson was also an amateur Jockey who owned two race horses himself, and could frequently be seen at the race-track riding his own horses. He rarely won, but was such a keen sportsman that he only went for the ride. Another of his pursuits was to go to the Serpentine in Hyde Park with his cronies on Christmas Day, to break the ice.

When he retired, it was said by the local fraternity, that the last bit of life in Rye Lane had died with him. This has indeed proved to be so.

Mr Warrener was a bookie's runner in the days before the

betting shops. In 1955 his work was quite illegal; he took bets while standing in a telephone kiosk, from people in public houses, or while standing on a street corner in Rye Lane. His job was to take the betting slips with the punters' money, carry them to the bookmaker in his office, then pay out the winners on the following day in the same illegal fashion.

His favourite place of business was the Hope public house in Rye Lane, where Mr Deveson was the landlord, but Mr Deveson turned a blind eye to his activities. After all, it was good for business; a person coming in to place a bet invariably bought a drink.

Mr Warrener, a Peckhamite, was a well-known friend of the police, and they would tip him off when it was time for them to make an arrest for betting, to give him time to find a stooge. The stooge, paid by the bookie to play the part of the runner, would be arrested, but not having been involved in this illegal activity before, appeared before the magistrate as a first offender. He would therefore only get a ten pound fine - which the bookie would pay - and the stooge would also be rewarded by the bookie for his stand-in part. Mr Warrener, having already been apprehended on several occasions by new over-zealous policemen, would have been labelled a frequent offender, would have got a much heavier fine; even a custodial sentence. Mr Warrener, of necessity, spent most of his life in public houses, and he was my first encounter with *delirium tremens,* the DTs, in general practice.

I was called to see him late one night in November 1956, when he was living in Fenwick Road. He was shivering, running a high temperature, was hallucinating, and had taken to his bed. He had a persistent cough, his sputum was rust-coloured, and there was no doubt in my mind after I had examined his chest that the poor fellow had acute lobar pneumonia.

I gave him an injection of penicillin, said that I would call on the following morning to see how he was and, if his condition had not deteriorated, give him another injection. I was quite happy with the nursing care; a friend whom I knew well was providing this for him. I explained to her that should she be at all concerned during the night to send for me and I would get him hospitalized.

On the following morning, when I called again to see him to give him his second jab, he recognized me, greeted me and sat up in bed. With staring hollow eyes, he then insisted that I raise my hat to the lovely girls, Beryl, Sybil, Frances, Marilyn, Dulcie and Cheryl, in various parts of his room. I looked at him speechless, to see whether he was joking; there were only two people in the room; one of them was me! He was certainly not joking! When he saw I was not making any great haste in raising my hat, he began to shout at me for not behaving like a gentleman. He became hysterical, and tried to get out of bed with the obvious intention of striking me. I didn't wait to be asked again; feeling like a blithering idiot, I raised my trilby hat to these imaginary creatures littered round his room. It was not the raising of my hat which made me feel so foolish; I was wondering whether on the previous night I had made the wrong diagnosis. I had never seen a patient with the DTs before and thought Mr Warrener had gone mad.

According to him, two girls were sitting on top of the wardrobe, and one of these girls was now giving me serious grounds for concern. As she was, in his fantasies, attempting to climb out of his open upstairs window, and he kept shouting to her not to do so, I was afraid he might get out of bed in an attempt to save her. He might then accidentally fall out of the window himself. To humour him, I ran to the wardrobe, grabbed hold of an imaginary pair of ankles and pulled them down. I performed an imaginary rescue on this girl, I have never felt such a fool in my whole life. I have never been much of an actor, but I certainly played an excellent part that morning, I fooled him. I then went to the window and closed it firmly with the excuse that it was impossible to examine anybody in such a cold room.

Suddenly, without warning, he started brushing his bed to sweep away the spiders, and even while I was examining him he kept stroking this imaginary cat. It cost me a good deal of patience in treating this chap. Trying to give a patient an injection in his arm when he suddenly decides to use his arm to push away an imaginary cat is no joke. After the injection he insisted that his room had become full of cats. As his nurse had now come into the room we had the farcical situation of a qualified doctor and a nurse shooing non-existent cats from his room. Anyone who did not know the situation and was passing by would have had us locked up as loonies. Rather surprisingly, he never complained there were mice or rats in his room: I had always been taught that a person who suffers from DTs always sees imaginary rodents.

The performance of raising my hat to his imaginary girls persisted on my visit to him that evening, also on the following morning, and it reached the stage when I was seriously considering breaking my tradition and leaving my hat in the car. I had managed to fix the window so that it could not be opened easily, but I wondered what other tests he would set me if I appeared in his room hatless. I never tempted the fates, and went to see him on every occasion with my hat perched firmly on my head, so that we could play out our little charade.

I visited him twice a day to give him penicillin

injections and to monitor his progress, but happily the penicillin worked quickly, his temperature dropped after the fourth injection, and his cough improved too. His delusions however persisted until I managed to convince the nurse that not only was penicillin necessary for his recovery, so too was a pint of Guinness.

He was given a pint of Guinness on my instructions one morning, and when I returned that evening he behaved normally. He recovered completely and lived another twenty years until, when in his seventies, he had another bout of pneumonia. This was so virulent he only lasted one day. This attack did not even give him time to mention cats, spiders or 'those lovely girls on top of the wardrobe'.

Harold Baker lived in Talfourd Road with his wife and family when I first had the fortune to meet him in 1954. He came to register his family on my medical list with a smile on his face and I can never remember that smile leaving his face until the day he died.

He and his wife and two children lived in the same house for thirty years, but after his wife died he found it much too big for him. His children had by this time married and left the area; not only did he find the house too large, he was lonely. To keep him company he grew a long beard. I used to joke with him, it was probably the occupants of his beard which now provided him with company; being a non-stop talker, he had an audience.

I contacted the social services over his problems and we managed after a great deal of effort to get him transferred to the sheltered accommodation unit on the North Peckham Estate. After all, he was seventy-eight years old when he was moved; he was not jumping any queues. His beard had by this time become even longer, but the pleasant smiling face, cheerful outgoing behaviour, could always be seen underneath the undergrowth. Having known him for so long had made our relationship a very close one; we were more than patient and doctor, we were the best of friends.

When he was eighty-one years of age and had been in sheltered accommodation for three years his adventure on the pedestrian crossing took place. Every year, since his retirement at sixty-five, he had spent the winter months in Southern Ireland with his friends, but now, eighty-one years old, had felt too old to go there in the winter: he was postponing his trip until June. He always went by boat; he said the crossing in the winter was too rough and exhausting for a man of his age and as the sea was smoother in June he would go then. It was an on-going joke between us about his relationship with the Southern Irish for whenever he returned, trouble would break out in Northern Ireland. He stirred things up. It was therefore only his age which explained why in January 1988 Harold was still in Peckham, not on a farm in Tipperary.

Harold was a betting man, loved the horses, and I had never, as I have already stated, seen Harold without a smile on his face, even when his daily bets had failed to provide him with one winner. The betting shop is a very welcoming place for an old man who is fond of a small wager, knows when to curb his passion, and not put his pension on a certainty – which comes last. It was not so very odd therefore, when Harold was found crossing Peckham Road on his way to the betting shop one mild January morning in 1988. He was making his way on a zebra crossing, at the rear of a line of children on their way from Goldsmith School: a policeman on duty at this crossing was monitoring their passage across the road when the accident occurred.

Harold, at the rear of the procession, with a paper in his hand and his forecasts in his pocket, was knocked down by a car which had not pulled up in time. He had not noticed the car approaching him. To be honest, when he related the story to me, his mind had not been on cars but on gee-gees. He lay on the ground screaming in agony. He had sustained as we learned later from the hospital reports, a fractured femur. His absence of a detailed knowledge of anatomy did not worry him at the time; all he knew was that he was suffering agonizing pain in his right hip joint. Not only was the pain so intense but it was magnified at the knowledge that he had been felled on a police-monitored crossing. He had felt so safe! He had done the same journey, with the same children, at the same time, dozens of times, in perfect safety.

The policeman was beside himself with fury at the driver of the car. It was a lady, and when Harold first saw her, she was standing in the road crying, hysterical, shaking with fright. She was sobbing so loudly, was so speechless that the policeman was having difficulty in getting information from her. Harold could see that the poor Bobby was getting more and more frustrated and losing patience. He was not being helped either by the crowd of inquisitive children who were giving advice to the young policeman as to how to conduct his enquiries. Harold also had to fend them off as they persistently tried to get him to get up.

A large crowd had gathered, the main road was blocked, long-distance lorry drivers from the Continent negotiating the Dover to London road through Peckham must have been cursing whoever it was causing this delay. It was a real pantomime, as he told me so himself. He would have enjoyed it, had he not been in so much pain.

The policeman was taking turns in shouting questions at him then at the driver of the car. Both were in a state of shock, and in no fit state to give him any answers. There was a crowd looking on too, as if ready to clap, when the policeman finished his questioning. The policeman had made up his mind that as Harold was old he was deaf too, and Harold's hearing suffered for days as a result of the policeman's assumption. The policeman would stand up to question the lady, then stoop down to bellow in poor Harold's ear.

When he related the story to me later, he burst out laughing. 'You know, doc, that copper was really making a hell of a racket.'

The cause of all the commotion, the driver of the car, had become by this time a gibbering idiot, and a chair from Kennedy's, the cooked meat shop, had to be brought out for her to sit down.

The impasse was finally resolved when an ambulance arrived. The two ambulancemen in it tried to pacify Harold. He screamed in agony when they tried to move him while the policeman, completely oblivious to his shrieking, continued to bellow in his ear. The pantomime finally ended when the ambulancemen managed to coax Harold onto a stretcher, and with klaxon sounding took him to hospital.

A few days after the accident, when Harold had recovered somewhat from the shock and his leg had been pinned, he checked the racing results of that day and the true significance of the events of that tragic day hit him. He had asked the sister of the ward whether it would be possible for her to get him a newspaper of the day he was admitted, any newspaper would do. She said she would try. That evening she had triumphantly returned with a copy of *The Daily Mirror*.

He had been on his way to the betting shop, not returning from it. His forecasts were still in his pocket. He had been unable to place his bets. He had done a five horse yankee, three of the horses running at odds of 9-1, and two horses at 8-1. Every one of the horses had won! Had he only reached the betting shop his winnings would have amounted to *£43,000* for his *50p* bet!

It was not to be: fortune was not to smile on him. I explained to him that it makes one believe in God. Had he won such a large sum of money at his advanced age, he would have become a lager lout, or a good-for-nothing layabout. He could even have become a capitalist of the worst possible kind. Providence had been kind to him, saved him from disaster at the hands of a lady.

The lady who had knocked him down was probably the bookie's wife. She had saved her husband from disaster too. He would never have believed he could have lost so much money for just a 50p bet. The odds against Harold winning had been so great that the bookie would not have bothered to lay the bet off, he would have covered it himself. On finding that Harold had won so much money with such an insignificant bet, he would almost certainly have shot himself. Not only had Harold himself been saved but another man's life had been saved too.

Harold was unperturbed during my explanation; he remained with the same smile on his face which had enchanted me for the thirty-four years of our acquaintance. He put his hand into his breast pocket, and took out a crumpled sheet of paper which he proudly showed to me. On it was written the names of the horses which would have made him a rich man.

The money would indeed not have helped Harold very much. About eighteen months after the accident he had a stroke which proved fatal.

11

Malingerers

Some short event often impinges itself in one's memory, even when the episode occurred nearly forty years ago.

Mrs Waite lived in Whateley Road, East Dulwich, in 1956, and suffered from severe osteoarthritis in both knees and ankles. She was a short, obese lady, weighed over twenty stone, a grumpy soul, who hated to smile, and whose life consisted of one long grumble. She was much too fat to be able to leave her upstairs sitting-room and come to the surgery so I had the unfortunate duty of having to visit her whenever she required any medical attention.

I never bothered to find out what had happened to her husband, but with her temperament he had either left her, or departed this life to escape her carping. She never had a good word to say about anyone and hated her brother-in-law Mr Gray, who was the most inoffensive soul. She despised her sister for marrying Mr Gray, and I lost count at the number of times she told me this. As far as I knew, Mrs Waite had not been blessed with children.

She was sixty-three years old and tethered to an armchair. She was so grossly obese it prevented her from moving about to do her housework or be ambulant. The thought of the effort required to move this hunk of flesh must just have been too great for her to contemplate such an enterprise.

To me she was a nightmare: at that particular time I was trying to be extra nice to all my patients, trying to build up a viable medical list, and I had only accepted her as a patient as a favour to her sister Mrs Gray who lived in Lyndhurst Way round the corner from the surgery. I really had not wanted to accept her; I had already been warned by Mr Gray what type of a lady his sister-in-law was, but his wife was a formidable lady too, and I did not want to offend her. I really had no choice. What could a young doctor do when he was making every effort to build up a practice?

Mrs Waite was a very forthright lady, as formidable as her sister when it came to accepting advice from a young doctor. She suffered repeated attacks of bronchitis which I attributed to her smoking, obesity and lack of movement, and I unfortunately became a frequent visitor to her house. Treating bronchitis in 1956 meant giving twice daily intramuscular injections of penicillin, and visiting a patient one does not like, twice daily, is not a pleasant way of spending one's time. To be told every time after I had given an injection that the training which I had received in medical school had really not been sufficient for me to give a decent jab did not endear herself to me either. To be perfectly frank I hated having to go and visit her. She even made me so manic at times I prayed that the penicillin would not work and she would receive a call from the good Lord. My prayers were never answered, the penicillin always worked.

I did my best to get her to lose weight. I gave her diets, prescribed appetite suppressant tablets – the benzedrine derivatives were in vogue at the time – all to no avail. She continued to assail me with her acid tongue; I was in her opinion useless. What use was I, she constantly reminded me, when I could not cure any of her many ailments?

It was obviously my fault that she was fat, she suffered so cruelly, and that she suffered repeated attacks of bronchitis. To add to her troubles, she told me so to my face, she had now the misfortune of being registered with a doctor who was completely incompetent. He did not care whether his patient recovered or not. In this latter statement she was correct, although I would never have dared to tell her so to her face.

In spite of all my efforts I really was no good; I had been unable to come up with the right prescription to get her weight down. In desperation, I told her there was only one way, to cut down on the number of meals she ate during the day. After much argument I plucked up courage, and actually told her to change her doctor unless she agreed to do so. For once in her life she had been answered back and the effect was stunning: she agreed to cut down on the number of meals she ate during the day from five to three.

She sent for me again, two weeks after agreeing to my weight reduction advice, and told me I was still useless. She was heavier than ever and intended to do as I had suggested, to change to a decent doctor who would cure her. While telling me all this, protesting that she had not eaten anything for fourteen days on my instructions, she devoured a whole two pound tin of Mackintosh's Quality Street, which was conveniently placed on the sideboard. She chewed, crunched, munched, sucked, talked and swallowed, all the time. I was hypnotized. It was like seeing a cement mixer being filled, but instead of depositing its contents, swallowing them. I would have been sick eating such an amount. I felt sick just by watching her. When I told her she was putting on her own fat by eating chocolates, she berated me for being more stupid than ever. She was no longer eating meals on my advice, she was famished and feeling faint. Now, I had the intention of starving her to death.

I had been persecuted enough and answered her back; we did not part the best of friends. She changed her doctor. I learned from Mrs Gray about three months after the change that her sister was not too happy with her new doctor and would like to change back to me. The Almighty however spared me this problem in the winter of 1959, he took her to him and became her new doctor, before she could transfer back to me.

☆ ☆ ☆

All doctors have patients whom they classify as nuisances, malingerers, time-wasters; in my time I have had nothing to complain about, I have had my fair share.

Mr Hempson (Anthony), a man in his early forties, lived in Nutbrook Street in 1964. Whenever I saw him I became distraught; he invariably brought on one of my attacks of migraine. He practically lived in my surgery. I was sick to death of the sight of him. He mentally tortured me, he persecuted me, and as I had no way of ridding myself of him I suffered, and continued to do so for ten long years.

He was short, about five foot nothing in height, and looked the same in width. He was round-faced, and it is an understatement to say that he was obese. He was broad shouldered, heavily built, over twenty stone in weight, and never smiled. However hard I tried I could never get a smile out of him, he never ever showed any emotion. His wife almost matched him in size and temperament – they say animals come in pairs! Thank God they were childless!

The problem with him was that he constantly found a hole to fall into or fall out of; a shop to fall into or out of. He was apparently being pushed into, or out of something by someone, all the time. He was either knocked down by a car, tripped up by, or hit by an overhanging branch of a tree. Trees would sprout out of the ground in the most unusual places just for the purpose of injuring poor Anthony, and protruding roots caused him years of agony, pain and distress.

He was a lover of water. Water caused him untold injuries, and with the weather in this country being on the moist side he revelled in it. Water mixed with earth equals mud, and what slipping and sliding could be had with this mixture! He worshipped it. Why not? It gave him a very good living, thank you very much.

Walls were another of his favourite hobbies. A wall would fall on him, jump out of its position to hinder his passage, suddenly appear out of thin air to injure him, but never enough to complete the job to my satisfaction! These were just a few of his favourite complaints: I was the unwilling listener and forced processor of these.

We shared a life of continuous litigation. Not a week went by without my receiving a letter demanding a report from one firm of solicitors or another, about one accident or another. He never used one firm of solicitors for his litigation, he used a different firm for each complaint. I never found out why; I would have thought he would naturally have saved money by using just one firm. Perhaps it was just to persecute me!

By using different firms of solicitors he confused me, and caused me all sorts of problems. Whenever I received a letter about one of his accidents, I was forced to waste my time checking through the records, to match up the accident and the date with the firm of solicitors. One firm would write to me about an arm injury he had sustained on one day, another firm would write about a similar injury he claimed he had sustained a few days later. He was always the victim, never, never, could he ever in any circumstances have been the offender. I soon learned his strategy.

He had learnt very quickly that almost all the defendants he threatened to take to court preferred to settle out of court rather than risk the expense of prolonged litigation. This way he made a comfortable living from his 'accidents'.

For example, following an accident to his ankle, he would present himself at my surgery requiring treatment. His ankle would be swollen and deformed, and had all the signs of a sprain or fracture. From his moans and groans when he presented himself to me you would have thought he had sustained a major heart attack. He would indeed have been suffering some pain, but probably thought if he had to earn the money, he had to act the part. On every occasion, I took the precaution of having the offending bone or joint X-rayed, so that he would not have the excuse of litigating against me too.

He would then ask me for certificates to prove he had suffered injuries, which I honestly could not refuse. He had definitely suffered an injury. To prove whether it had been sustained wilfully or accidentally was impossible. There was no way any doctor could have stood in the witness box to prove that the accident he had suffered was self-inflicted. I was only giving him a certificate for an injury he had suffered not giving an opinion as to how it was caused.

He would on leaving me go to a firm of solicitors with my certificate to commence proceedings against the offending party. The firm he had chosen to represent him for that particular case would state to the offending party that their client would be prepared for the claim to be settled out of court – providing of course the damages were sufficiently rewarding.

He was astute, he had plenty of experience, obviously knew how much to ask without the defence being prepared to contest the amount in court. The local council did prepare a defence to one of his claims when he tripped over a loose paving stone in Blenheim Grove. This is where Anthony's experience told; he had chosen the right stone. This paving stone had been reported as faulty by someone else who had written to the council complaining about it, but had not been injured; so was making no claim. Whether the writer of the letter and Anthony were in collusion I never found out, but the council settled out of court and repaired the fault rather than fight a losing suit.

This agony of mine went on for some years. He once absent-mindedly scratched himself on a tree in the front garden of my surgery. He had obviously forgotten where he was, that I knew his game. When he came to complain to me, all he got for his pains was in injection against lockjaw, a reprimand to watch where he walked in future, and a green form to take to the optician – for an eye test.

One of his favourite stunts, I had written many reports on his accidents of this type to his solicitors, was to stand up in a bus, just as it was going to stop. He would then hope the driver would slam the brakes on so quickly that the bus would lurch forward. The more violent the lurch, the better!

If the lurch was sudden and violent, he was in clover. He would arrive at my surgery immediately afterwards as an emergency with some injury or another. His arm would ache for weeks. I lost count at the number of whiplash injuries recorded in my medical records as a result of one of these lurches. Unfortunately, although lawyers may have different opinions, it is not always easy for a doctor to diagnose whether a patient has a whiplash injury or strained ligaments in the spine as a result of an accident. It is of course possible these symptoms preceded the accident, but to prove it is impossible.

Fortune favoured me at last; he decided to move away from Nutbrook Street to the Forest Hill area. I plucked up courage and told him that as both he and his wife were now residing outside my catchment area, they would have to find a new doctor. This was in 1974.

I had suffered ten years of misery and hell, but had previously never had the guts to tell him to find another doctor. His moving gave me the excuse I had prayed for, and the couple actually changed their doctor. I saw them once or twice afterwards whilst out shopping in Rye Lane, but purposely crossed the road before we could meet.

Five years later, I read about his last escapade in the local paper. He had fallen down the stairs of a double-decker bus in Rye Lane. The bus had suddenly made an emergency stop to avoid hitting a pedestrian; on this occasion his fall had been ill-timed. He fell out of the bus into the road and sustained a fractured skull. He died in the ambulance on the way to hospital.

☆ ☆ ☆

Anthony Lovelock was a man in his early fifties, pot-bellied, round-shouldered, grey-haired and balding, who appeared much older than his stated age and caused me all sorts of problems in May 1958.

When he did not return from work at his usual time at

six o'clock one Friday evening his wife became anxious and phoned his workplace. He worked as a bus inspector, his base was at New Cross, and she was told that he had left work at the usual time. She was made more anxious by the fact that Anthony was an introvert, he never went out without her, never visited pubs, and from the day of their marriage had always come straight home from work. He was thought by his mates at the garage to have gone straight home so when midnight came and no Anthony she phoned the police. The police were unable to help, they promised Mrs Lovelock to keep a look out, but this was probably said to her just to allay her anxiety.

Help finally came, when a middle-aged lady walking a dog through Greenwich Park on the following Tuesday went to the Greenwich police and reported a suspicious character. In her opinion this chap was either a pervert, a child molester, or a raving lunatic. Whenever she now passed, he made funny faces, stuck his tongue out, and fiddled with the fly buttons on his trousers. He appeared to her to have been sitting on the same bench for two days; he had no beard when she had first noticed him, now he did. He had looked quite presentable when first seen by her, he had winked, smiled and whistled after her. She had been flattered at the time, this is why she had particularly noticed him. No one had apparently taken any notice of her for years, and she had therefore deliberately gone past the bench to see her 'suitor' afterwards. Since he had now become dirty and unkempt, no longer a person with whom one would wish to be associated, she had reported his behaviour to the authorities. The police went to investigate the suspicious character on the park bench, and although Anthony could, or would not tell them who he was, they had found ample papers in his pockets to identify him. They brought him home.

Anthony had been missing four days when the police asked me to call at his home in Parkstone Road. The time was 8 p.m., I had finished surgery, I therefore had ample time to examine him thoroughly. I cannot remember whether it had rained during his escapade, no mention of this can be found in my notes, but I found examining him a most unpleasant experience – he stank. The stench from his clothes hit my nostrils even before I entered the room, and I had to use every artifice in my personality to prevent his wife from seeing me retching.

Anthony appeared to have amnesia. Although I had previously seen him on many occasions, he did not appear to recognize me, nor did he appear to recognize his wife or mother-in-law. Maybe his non-recognition was from choice; his mother-in-law lived with them.

As I could find no organic cause for his symptoms I called in a neurologist. The neurologist thought that Anthony might have had a brain haemorrhage, his symptoms at the time appeared to fit in with this theory, but as this man had no history of high blood pressure we were both unconvinced of this diagnosis. Of one thing the neurologist was certain: he did not want Anthony as one of his patients; he was passed back to me to deal with.

Anthony's behaviour was odd; apart from the fact he did not know who he was, he also appeared to be disorientated in time and place. Now safely in his home environment, he ate, drank and slept. Sleep was unavoidable, I kept him heavily sedated; I did not want him wandering off again before I had made some sort of a diagnosis. I followed his progress for a week, but he still developed no signs of any organic disorder which I could recognize. As his behaviour had not improved, his wife was having to act as a prison warder, to prevent him leaving the house and getting lost again. I now referred him for a psychiatric opinion.

The psychiatrist came, chatted to Anthony, Anthony's wife, the mother-in-law, finally me: he then made the diagnosis – Anthony was suffering from an acute confusional state. His diagnosis was brilliant, he had actually put a name on what Anthony was suffering from. Anthony's wife was unimpressed, so was I.

'I could have told him what my husband was suffering from on the phone,' she said.

After several visits to the psychiatrist he appeared to be in the same condition as when first found. No one appeared to have the answer. The only solution which was now being seriously considered was to have the poor chap admitted to a mental institution.

His mother-in-law, after her husband's death two years previously, had come down from Lincoln to live with the couple. She had been happy until Anthony had his 'turn', but now could not take the pressure of her son-in-law's behaviour. He had never been a bad son-in-law, but then her daughter had been able to devote all her time to her: the daughter now had her hands full, mother-in-law was having to play second fiddle. She had therefore decided to return to Lincoln and live with another daughter.

She left, and Anthony appeared to make a miraculous recovery. To be fair, it still took a week or so for his amnesia to resolve completely, but resolve it did.

Whether he had a genuine cerebral vascular leak which had damaged his brain or mother-in-lawitis, I have never been too sure.

12

Slices of Life

Doctor Blank (Merton), had been practising single-handed in Choumert Road before becoming one of the founder members of our group practice. He had first come down to London from Southport, to succeed Dr Mackay, who had a surgery in Choumert Road. Poor Dr Mackay had died while attending a patient, and I was informed at the time that the patient had been annoyed at not having received a sick note before the 'deadly event' had taken place.

Merton was a loveable eccentric. He was blunt to the extreme, an impish man, with an infectious laugh. Many of his eccentricities could have been laid at the door of his very poor unbringing, for he would go to extraordinary lengths to save money. He just could not get used to spending money, even when he eventually had some, and was in a position to do so.

Medicine was not his first career, he was an industrial chemist, having obtained a first-class honours degree from Manchester University. His job took him to Paris for a year or so, and he took the opportunity of learning to speak French. When he returned, his employers put him on the night shift, whereupon he handed in his notice. On failing to secure new employment after six months, he went back to Manchester University to seek advice, and it was on their suggestion that he took up a medical career.

He was a very bright young fellow and qualified easily. He was an excellent diagnostician, a really excellent doctor, but lacked the bedside manner. Many patients were terrified of him; unless they were really ill he had no time for them. In fact, if a patient was given a certificate by him to stay away from work, it meant that they were at death's door!

His economical behaviour, although frequently commented on by the other doctors and staff, was not exclusively devoted to work, it was even more stringently applied at home. Merton's wife Lena used to say to the children, 'You tell me what you want, and I will tell you how to manage without it.'

She knew that unless something was essential, Merton would not countenance its purchase.

Merton appropriated Lena's car when they met; she lost the use of it, and eventually her licence expired. She was then forced to use buses to do her shopping and visit her friends. Merton made two stipulations when he bought a new car:

1) It had to have a starting handle: he used to crank up his engine to save the battery, every morning.

2) It must not have an automatic choke, this would lead to slight wastage of petrol.

When his son first learned to drive, Merton sold him his car second-hand, at what his son believed to be the second-hand market price. When his son traded it in for a new one after passing the driving test, he found his father had overcharged him for it!

Running a car has always been an expensive item. Merton, who was forced to have one by virtue of his work, devised driving economies. When he wanted to signal, he declined to use the indicators, prior to that trafficators, because at some point he would have to replace a bulb. Instead, he would wind down the window and give hand signals. It might have been snowing, the passengers shivering from cold from the open window, it did not make a scrap of difference.

Whenever he did some gardening or cleaned the car, he would never use a belt to hold his trousers up, he made do with an old tie. After cleaning the car, he would go inside the house to get a member of the family help him push it back into the garage. He would not dream of starting it by using the starter motor – this would have led to some drain in the battery.

He was never seen to use a handkerchief, only tissues, usually those which came with boxes of apples. He would polish his shoes after every wear, so managed to make them last indefinitely. When his shoe laces broke, rather than buy new ones he made them do by tying the broken ends.

One of the many economies which he forced on his family was not to use more than two inches of water for bathing. Even today, when his son manages to indulge himself in a bath which is as much as half full, he is left with a feeling of guilt. He used to wash his hair (what little he had) with soap which was much cheaper than shampoo. He was meticulous in dental care, but instead of buying tooth-picks, he used his penknife to whittle down old matches which he found.

His son had to keep a log of his phone calls, and pay for them when the quarterly bill arrived. When one day he telephoned the surgery to speak to his father, Merton was overheard to say, 'Where are you speaking from? – my house? – get off the phone! I will speak to you later.'

He would not wear socks and many are the stories which have been told to me of this peculiarity. At one meeting of the committee of the St Mary's Road General Practitioners' Centre I was met by the acid remarks of one member, 'Can't you afford to pay your partner enough to allow him to buy himself a pair of socks?'

This of course was followed by shrieks of laughter at my expense. I was really not too embarrassed; all the doctors on the committee knew of his behaviour. Patients would take great delight in telling me that they had seen Dr Blank, walking in Ruskin Park, whatever the weather, reading a newspaper, with torn trousers and slippers, and without a hat or coat.

One day, just as I was about to commence an evening surgery, a patient whom I knew very well, rushed in to tell me he had just seen a 'poofter' changing his trousers round the corner in his car, outside the Albert public house. He was amused, wanted me to join in the fun.

'It shouldn't be allowed, should be reported,' he said.

I went with him to see this remarkable event, but was disappointed to find that it was just Merton changing into smart trousers which he wore in the surgery from the threadbare ones he used when he travelled in his car. He was only being economical!

The staff in the surgery loved, understood and had a great affection for him. They looked forward each day to another Dr Blank episode: he had this great ability, which is so extremely rare, of being able to laugh at himself. He would throw his head back, laugh uproariously even though he himself was the victim, the object of the merriment. One of their many pranks was to offer him a sweet, which he never refused, and leave the sweets in a bag on a desk. When he thought they were not looking, with his back to the sweets, he would thrust his hand into the bag and take some more. Someone would then go to take a sweet and remark, 'Some thieving ratbag has taken more than his fair share.'

At a post-graduate lecture at the General Practitioners' centre one Thursday afternoon, the sister in charge called me out of the room to have a quiet word with me. Approaching me with embarrassment she said, 'Do you know your partner, Dr Blank, takes biscuits during the tea interval, hides them in his pocket, then eats them in the toilet like a naughty boy?'

She told me the story in a loud whisper, for my ears only, not to be heard, even by the walls. She was so embarrassed! As she concluded her recital I fell about laughing, and her attitude changed completely. She realized it was nothing which really gave me concern, nothing which would cause disharmony in our group practice by her disclosure, nothing to cause a break-up. In between peals of laughter, I promised to buy her a packet of biscuits to replace the loss. When she saw my reaction she could not contain herself, she too saw the funny side of her story, she too burst into peals of laughter. She had never come across a situation like this before – neither had I.

His relationship with Nellie the housekeeper who lived in the practice premises gave us in the practice many a chuckle. Merton was an orthodox Jew. Although he would do surgery on Friday evening in the winter when the sabbath had already commenced, he would not switch the lights on or off. After doing his surgery, he would shout, 'NELLIE! *Shabbos!* Lights!'

She would shuffle down to do his bidding.

When the garden gate broke down, he would shout, 'NELLIE! Gate!'

She would shuffle down, this time with hammer and nails.

She grew fruit in the garden. He would wait until they became ripe, then while her back was turned, would steal them. The only remark from her when she went to pick her fruit would be, 'That thieving ratbag has pinched my fruit again!'

He was so obsessed with cost cutting, even in the surgery, that he would switch my light and fire off the moment I left my consulting room. He would accept my explanation that his actions were not cost-effective; fluorescent lights were better left on, rather than switched on and off incessantly, but this did not deter him. Old habits die hard; he continued to switch my lights and fire off.

We had many a tussle over his behaviour, perhaps he over mine, but we always parted the best of friends. I must admit I was fond of him, he was a character, but a lovable one. Although he had the name of being mean and miserly, he was the most liberal host when I was a guest in his home.

I had the privilege of being his general practitioner and I was very saddened, when the heart trouble which had shortened his work pattern in the latter years finally ended his life – at much too early an age.

☆ ☆ ☆

The prize of being a long-serving general practitioner in the same practice is that I now have the opportunity of treating the great-great grandchildren of some of my original patients.

One family with whom I have been associated both as doctor and friend is the Perry family, and four generations of this family are still patients of this practice. Mrs Clark, a sweet lady in her late seventies I still treat, and the reason I have chosen her mother as the subject of this story is that I remember her mother so well.

Mrs Perry was a pleasant, extremely fat lady, a smile

perpetually on her face, blessed with a fabulous sense of humour. She was so obese – well over twenty stone in fact – I can only ever remember seeing her seated. I must however admit that I only became her doctor at the tail end of her life. Her ulcerated legs gave cause for concern, my visits to her home were of necessity frequent, but I never left her home without having had a good laugh. Evidently, her weight problem had been with her all her life for all her stories related to this fact. This remarkable feat at being able to joke about her own disability is the reason I remember her so well, even though the incidents she related took place over sixty years ago.

Of the many stories which she related about her problems, the one I love best is the one about her adventure on a very busy Saturday afternoon in the Millwall football ground. She was an avid Millwall fan; although she could not afford to travel to their away matches she attended all their matches at the Den – would have died rather than miss one.

One Saturday afternoon, on the day of the special cup match, she went to the ground early, as she wanted to get a good standing position. Being fat, she liked to have something to hold on to. Next to one of the intermittent poles, which supported the stand seats of the more wealthy patrons, was her favourite position. She had walked to the ground from her home in Marmont Road, which was a distance of one mile, and was feeling just that little bit tired.

On this occasion, tiredness and excitement merged, and she did not pay too much attention to detail in trying to get through the turnstile. She always had to be extra careful as to how to get through the turnstile, and had to manoeuvre her fat body sideways to go through. As she had performed the feat dozens of times it had become second nature to her, she did it automatically – today she forgot!

It was a cup match, other Millwall fans had noted the same fact, and had turned up early too. There was a crowd entering the ground, there was some pushing and shoving and the ground was filling up. As she stood in the queue waiting her turn at the paying-in desk her excitement boiled over, she wondered whether she would be lucky enough to get a good position to see the match. Getting through the turnstile was the last thing in her mind!

She paid her money at the kiosk and made a fatal mistake: she attempted to get into the ground as she had seen everyone else do, she tried to go through the turnstile frontways. No go! She now tried to manoeuvre herself, moved from side to side, trying to get through sideways, but this only allowed the turnstile to get an even firmer grip on her body. She had committed the mortal sin of trying to enter the turnstile as everyone else did, and the turnstile was not going to let her forget it. She just could not budge her bulk.

The road was closed, she was the blockage, and having placed herself in such a position, she was never going to be removed without pieces being removed from her body. In the case of a baby who is having problems being delivered, forceps are used, no manufacturer however had yet had the foresight to produce a forceps large enough to extract a twenty plus stone woman from a turnstile.

She was stuck! Not only was she firmly and truly fastened in the contraption, she was almost hysterical from the considerable amount of discomfort of being positioned in this manner: also from the ministrations of the frustrated crowd waiting behind her. The crowd waiting to get in had also turned up early, hoping to get good positions. They were being thwarted by this immovable object who was determined to prevent them from doing so. They tried to do the impossible, to push her through!

The kiosk attendant had been on duty many Saturday afternoons when Mrs Perry had gone through his turnstile, and realized at once that there was going to be no solution to her mistake - except by the use of force. He had used initiative and called the fire brigade. The firemen arrived, removed the turnstile, and cut her free. A tremendous cheer went up from the crowd behind her when she was finally allowed into the ground, without having to pay the normal entrance fee. She was also rewarded by being given a free season ticket to the stand. It was cheaper for the club to provide her with this luxury, than to watch her have a return match with the turnstile.

☆ ☆ ☆

They were the lucky pair who had won a prize! The top prize in the Top Rank Bingo Club in 1977 which was a trip for two to Monte Carlo. Everyone was envious, it was not surprising, who would not be envious of a couple who had struck so lucky just by playing bingo?

Mr Patrick O'Flaherty worked for a firm of contractors as a sprinkler fitter, fitting sprinklers in large buildings for use in case of fire; he had however never earned enough to be able to afford such a trip as this prize offered. His work had demanded that he travelled the length and breadth of this country, never abroad. He had indeed worked in the airport at odd times for over twenty years installing sprinklers in the shops and in the new hangars there, but the only occasion he had left these shores was a trip to Ireland - by boat. He had never flown, never actually been in an aircraft; the thought of flying terrified him.

We now had a problem. The prize, a week in Monte Carlo, was by air. Although they were overjoyed at winning, Patrick spent sleepless nights worrying about the journey to Monte Carlo. As Mrs O'Flaherty had flown before, she had been on a pilgrimage to Lourdes, she did not have the same fears.

Patrick was persuaded by me and his wife he had nothing to worry about, he was a religious man, and the prize had obviously been sent as a gift from heaven. Our powers of persuasion overcame his reluctance; he duly arrived at the airport terminal at the appointed time and took his seat on the aircraft.

The plane took off dead on time and the flight was uneventful, until they reached Nice. He had by this time begun to feel that his fears had been unfounded. The plane had not met any turbulence at all. The food was good and the drink was plentiful. The air hostesses besides being very pretty were very helpful; in fact he was glad he came, he was actually enjoying himself!

Suddenly, when it had almost reached its destination, when over Nice the plane fell 12,000 feet and became depressurized. It had just fallen out of the sky without warning or meeting any turbulence.

Mrs Nancy O'Flaherty, a religious Catholic, calmly took out her holy water from her handbag and, walking down the gangway, made a blessing as she sprinkled it over the passengers. Patrick meanwhile had collapsed in his seat, but she did not pay much attention to his condition. She knew his fear of flying, thought he was just suffering from shock, so continued her religious ministrations. On review, his attack was not only due to shock, he had also suffered his first mild CVA (stroke).

The plane, in order to avoid being stranded in Monte

Carlo and having to pay airport fees before being repaired, limped back to Luton where it made an emergency landing. They were offered another flight to Monte Carlo, but refused. They had suffered enough! No amount of persuasion on behalf of the airline could make them board another plane even though all the other passengers had done so. They returned home.

Poor Mr O'Flaherty was in bed for six weeks after this flight, was unable to swallow properly, lost two stones in weight and to be honest has never been right since. He recovered enough however after a few months to stagger back to work, but only managed to do so until 1981 when he had another stroke. He has had several small ones since: although he has always appeared to recover physically after his strokes, each one has left him a little more mentally disturbed. After each stroke he has become more neurotic, hypochondriacal, and has taken up a lot of my time in treating his symptoms.

It appears to be a fact of life that misfortune, illness or conversely, luck once it appears, continues to strike the same person over and over again. Misfortune having once shown its ugly face, certainly continued to dog poor Mr O'Flaherty. He bought a bottle of his favourite beer one day, put it down by the side of his favourite chair when it exploded and injured him. He claimed against the company and his claim was not contested, it was settled out of court – they must have heard of Patrick's luck!

This injury however just deepened his depression. He had never been the same man after his flight to Monte Carlo and the bottle incident had not helped matters. He was now unable to concentrate for any length of time, completely lacked motivation and became even more hypochondriacal. He stayed in bed most of the day and Mrs O'Flaherty could not get him out of the house except to take the dog for a walk; this, once a day, then only for ten minutes. True, he got up for breakfast, but after eating it, went to bed. He got up for lunch at 12.30 p.m., ate his lunch, then went back again to bed. Tea was the only exception to the routine. He got up for tea at 4.30 p.m., and instead of going straight to bed afterwards took the dog out for a ten minute walk; then went to bed. He got up again at 8 p.m., had his supper, and went to bed. He had become a walking cabbage.

This cycle was repeated for a year before I was able to persuade the O'Flahertys that my knowledge of treating a man with these symptoms was minimal, that psychiatric help should be requested. They finally agreed, and he has attended for sessions with the psychiatrist for some years, but the psychiatrist has not appeared to be able to help him very much more than I did.

His last visit was in November 1990, when the psychiatrist explained that due to the problems with the hospital budget, the hospital was unable to meet its commitments. It was therefore having to cut down on outpatients' clinics. Patrick had in any event only been attending for social reasons; it had been somewhere to go, the only way we knew of getting him out of the house. For some time his symptoms had not improved at all, and he knew that the psychiatrist was aware of this.

He therefore understood the implications of the psychiatrist's remarks when he said, 'We have been unable to do very much for you Mr O'Flaherty, in all the years we have been treating you, perhaps your GP would have been just as good!'

Patrick did not answer.

The psychiatrist then looked into his eyes and without batting an eyelid said, 'Have you ever contemplated suicide?'

'Not until you just mentioned it,' Patrick replied.

I am now landed with him – but will cope – our relationship has extended over a period of thirty-five years.

The moral of this story is, 'If you have to win at bingo, for God's sake don't win the top prize.'

☆ ☆ ☆

Patients often have strange ideas of death and dying: when Mrs Wheeler's daughter sent for me in 1965 requesting a visit to her mother saying that she was dying, I was not terribly worried. The daughter phoned at 8.30 a.m. asking for an urgent visit, her mother might not last until the end of my morning surgery.

Mrs Wheeler was an eighty-six years old lady, and was being treated by me at the time for an ulcerated stomach. She had been up and about when I had last seen her in the previous week and I had not at that time expected such a drastic change in her condition. The message I had received requesting the visit was that Mrs Wheeler has passed a black motion, has taken to her bed feeling faint, and is now too weak to leave it.

I had already had enough experience to realize that in old age anything can be expected to occur suddenly, but I knew from the past record of this family that nothing really serious had occurred. On the one occasion when something serious had really happened, the daughter had propelled herself down the road to knock at my door. Nevertheless, there was always the possibility the old lady's ulcer had burst, or she had had a haemorrhage. Rather than give myself an ulcer from worrying, I decided to ease my conscience and visit her before I started morning surgery.

The old lady was lying in bed in a white nightdress, everything in the room was white, ghostly, even the curtains had an eerie look about them. Mrs Wheeler however appeared to be cheerful, she was quite delighted to see me. She told me, and her daughter agreed with her, that as she had passed a black motion, she was now waiting for the angel of death to call. The black motion had been a sign to her mortification had set in: her mother who had died at the age of ninety-seven had told her this. It obviously had in her particular case commenced in her bowels, and as it was the first sign of death she had thought it right and proper I should be notified. She was now waiting for the process of mortification to continue. There was no doubt in her mind, I had only been asked to call to verify the fact, perhaps as a second opinion. She had kept the stool as evidence.

There must have been some irritation in my behaviour which showed, for the daughter called me aside to explain the real reason for the urgency. She wanted to know from me how many hours the old lady had left. She was as sure as her mother was that the end was nigh, but wondered whether she would have time to do her morning shopping before the angel of death called.

This practice has had some strange men who wanted a sex change, to become women, but the oddest of them all was a chap called John who insisted on being called Jaynee Lee. John, alias Jaynee Lee wanted his sex change when he was forty-six years old. One of my partners who was first asked to deal with his problem remarked to him, 'You must be crazy to want a sex change at your age, you will be right in the middle of your change!'

My partner was right, John was crazy. John, refused help from my partner, transferred his attention to me and proceeded to drive me mad to get a sex change. He wanted to be a woman, dressed like one, and insisted that he required to take the contraceptive pill. It was no use my trying to persuade him that at the age of forty-six he (she) would be very unlikely to conceive. Jaynee Lee wanted the pill even though he (she) did not have a partner, and to keep him quiet I had no alternative but to acquiesce. I prescribed the pill for him, also tablets for his nerves. Anything to get him off my back. He used to waste my time with utter nonsense, I dreaded a consultation with him, he was the ultimate in looniness. The psychiatrist to whom I referred him was of little help, he prescribed antidepressants for him, counselled him about his aberration, but sent him back to me for treatment.

John (Jaynee Lee), would insist on seeing me whenever he read in the newspapers that the pill had side effects, or a patient had blamed the pill for her illness. The newspapers live by sensational reporting. If a girl on the pill develops a hump in Alaska it makes headlines, and if she is taking the contraceptive pill it obviously has to be the cause. He would avidly read the newspapers trying to find in them any new information relating to the pill or sex change, and if he did, I was in for a restless and troublesome fortnight.

I had the dubious task in persuading him that he would come to no harm on the pill which was being prescribed for him, but he did cause me to box clever on one occasion. The newspaper which he read ran a long medical report one day linking cancer of the cervix (neck of the womb) with the contraceptive pill, and he came to see me in a terrible state. He complained of feeling tired, pain in the lower part of his abdomen, pain in passing water, and demanded to know whether the pill which was being prescribed could cause him to have cancer of the womb. Not having a womb stunned my perception of his problem, and caused me to think for a moment. When I realized he was daft to ask such a question, I could honestly reassure him that his 'female' parts were not in jeopardy!

Jaynee Lee had a face which always looked as if it needed a shave, and to cover the stubble he added a thick layer of powder. He wore lipstick, grew his hair long and plaited it, but forgot he had a moustache! High heels, long plastic boots, mini skirt displaying hairy legs and a shoulder bag completed his ensemble.

The Almighty appeared to side with me about Jaynee Lee; he too disapproved of his attempts to become a woman and he gave him a deep bass voice. When this apparition called Jaynee Lee spoke, anyone who had never previously met him listened in stunned silence.

I will always remember the first occasion that we met. It was in 1978, when he was sitting on the front doorstep of the surgery waiting for the door to be opened and for the afternoon surgery to begin, but clearly did not see the female part of this creature, just noted his moustache. In my nonsensical way, I called out loudly, 'Good afternoon, sir.'

He jumped up as if he had been shot; I thought he was going to hit me; his violent reaction caused me to glance again.

This time without batting an eyelid I said, 'Sorry, good afternoon, madam.'

He grinned and sat down, satisfied that I had established his true gender.

Jaynee Lee was a chatterbox, a non-stop talker, who would sit in the waiting-room chatting to the other patients while waiting to see me. The patients in the room would sit uncomfortably, making every effort to ignore him. I opened my surgery door one day and saw this little black boy who was usually a nuisance in the waiting-room sitting quietly bolt upright with his mouth wide open. Whenever this boy had previously come to the surgery I had quickly been made aware of his presence.

The boy, now quiet as a dormouse, was sitting on the right of the room as I opened my door and I just had to follow the boy's eyes to see what had caused his deafening silence. He was looking at this strange creature in a mini skirt and hairy legs: the boy's eyes were popping out of his head. He was holding his mother's hand very tightly, wondering what the strange animal was. John was talking to the boy, but the boy was too terrified to answer.

Unfortunately, looking so strange and behaving so oddly John became a victim of scavengers and layabouts who tormented him, and made his life an absolute misery. He was to these tormentors an object of ridicule, and they wrote graffiti on the front door of his flat in Kirkwood Road so that passers-by should know who the occupant was. They had also put a notice in white paint on his front door which read 'the crazy man or woman lives here - please knock hard'.

Finally, drug abusers moved into his flat. When I had to visit him one day for a chest infection, he was an asthmatic, I found that the flat had been turned into a squalid dump. It had nine teenage residents, black and white, all doped up to the eyeballs, lying about the place. He was apparently unable to rid himself of his friends (tormentors) by normal means and in desperation decided to burn his flat down.

One day, his neighbours smelled burning and saw the passageway of the block filled with smoke so they called the Fire Brigade. When they arrived, they found John quietly sitting on the steps to the entrance of the block rolling a cigarette and humming to himself. He had finally flipped, and was sent into a mental institution.

My partner was right, John should never have wished to change his sex in the middle of the 'change'. Sadly, I learned later he had died during an attack of asthma.

It was a lovely warm sunny May morning in 1962, when I was asked to visit Mr Raymond Wellington, in Copleston Road. The reason given for the request was that he was not feeling too well; not ill enough to go to bed, but not well enough to come to the surgery. He was short of breath, had indigestion, felt sick, and had vomited twice. The message as passed to me also gave the diagnosis – he had eaten a ham sandwich for breakfast and it had upset his stomach. The visit I was informed could wait until after the morning surgery, there was no urgency.

I was already attending the Wellington sisters and two brothers with their various complaints; it could be said that I knew this family very well. It was a strange family. There were seven Wellingtons in all, four brothers and three sisters. Three brothers and three sisters all in their late fifties or early sixties, all unmarried, lived in the same house in Copleston Road. The seventh Wellington, the eldest brother, was the exception. He was married, lived in a village in Kent, and was the only member of the family not a patient of mine.

The brother to whom I had been called had a history of heart trouble, he had suffered from rheumatic fever as a child which had damaged his heart, but he had never had a heart attack. The technology we have today was not available in 1962, and the severity of his heart disease had been impossible to evaluate.

Raymond Wellington was a short stocky man, fifty-eight years old, and when I arrived at the house at 11.30 a.m. on that sunny morning he was sitting in an armchair in the lounge with his right arm firmly clutching his breastbone. He complained of a feeling of tightness in his chest, like a tight band going round his chest. He could not stop belching. He was certain it was indigestion, but while talking to me, giving me his history and describing his symptoms, his face became ashen, his lips paled and he began fighting for breath. His head fell forward, he collapsed in the chair and lost consciousness. I made every effort to resuscitate him. I even gave him an injection of adrenaline directly into his heart, but it was useless. A post mortem later revealed he had suffered a massive heart attack.

I called an ambulance, but when the attendants found the chap was dead and that I was prepared to sign the death certificate, they refused to take the body away. They were only allowed to take live bodies away they said, not dead ones. I packed up my medical bag, told the sisters to get in touch with Mays in Rye Lane, the local undertakers, and prepared to leave. I explained to one of the sisters that there would be no trouble in my issuing a death certificate. I had attended Raymond before death, and was quite satisfied that the cause of death was due to coronary thrombosis. If she came to the surgery later on, after I had completed my visits, I would give her a death certificate to take to the registrar; his offices I explained to her were situated opposite the town hall in Peckham Road.

Another sister then approached me and asked me to see James, another brother, who was in one of the bedrooms upstairs not feeling too well. He had not been in the lounge when I arrived, he had not wanted to see me for some reason, but had become so distressed on hearing of his brother's death that he had collapsed on the bed. I ran up the stairs like a hare – I was young at the time – but I was already too late! He was lying face upwards on the bed still, completely lifeless, his lips deep purple, frothy blood slowly oozing from the side of his mouth. He had obviously been dead for some minutes. There was nothing I could do.

To say this double tragedy shocked me would be an understatement. I went downstairs with two of the sisters, numbed, shattered! I had never had two deaths in one house at the same time before. Thank heavens in forty years this performance has never been repeated.

I sat with the three sisters in the back kitchen-cum-dining-room for some minutes, discussing what best to do in this extraordinary situation. Now that two brothers had decided to depart on the same day in what appeared to be in the same fashion, I suggested that in the circumstances it would be best for me to refer both deaths to the coroner. They were very reluctant. I would save them a good deal of aggravation and pain if I issued death certificates.

'After all, you have been treating both of them for heart trouble,' said one of the sisters, 'ask Harold, he will tell you how ill they were.'

Harold was the third brother in the house. He had gone to the toilet on my arrival. I had now been in the house for over an hour and we all suddenly looked at one another, stunned into silence. There were four of us in that room, no Harold.

The three sisters, for the one and only time, looked as if their world had collapsed. Indeed, it already had. The eldest sister was fat, round-faced, rosy-cheeked, very stout, staid and unflappable. The second sister, taller, very much thinner, suffered from multiple sclerosis, was in a wheelchair and got about with difficulty. She had remained downstairs whilst we dealt with the second brother, and the trauma of losing two brothers had not yet affected her quite as much as her sisters; she had only seen one of the brothers dead.

The third sister, of medium height, thin-faced, who never smiled, was a multi-symptomatic lady. She was in a state of constant anxiety, a complete bag of nerves, her hands shook all the time. She came to see me in the surgery every couple of days with a new symptom. I had not as yet found anything seriously wrong with her, I believe she would have been happier if I had. Nevertheless, we had a very friendly relationship. Even if she admitted my treatment had not cured her of her symptoms, she bore me no malice. She did not want to be cured; she enjoyed living with ill health.

They lived in a very old rambling house, as I had not seen Harry since coming into the house I naturally thought he was still in the toilet. I didn't want to ask questions, ran through the kitchen, round the back of the house and outside to the toilet.

The door was open, the toilet was empty – no Harry.

I walked back into the dining-room looking extremely puzzled and asked them if Harry could possibly have gone out before I arrived.

'We told you, he is in the toilet,' they answered in unison.

'We had an inside toilet and bathroom put in upstairs last year. It's at the side of the front bedroom.'

I ran upstairs and tried the toilet door. It was locked. I shouted, 'Harry! Harry!' hoping that he would open the door. There was no reply.

The two sisters who were mobile had by this time joined me upstairs, but the fat one had arrived in such a state of breathlessness that I thought that more resuscitation was going to be required. I now began to bang on the toilet door, and as this brought no response from inside, put my ear to the door to see whether I could hear movement. I could hear nothing. I then asked them if they would give me permission to force the lock.

The unflappable sister, the one who was always in charge, the eldest sister, the fat one, the one who managed the housekeeping, had by this time recovered from her climb up the stairs, now appeared as unperturbed as ever and gave her permission. I broke the door down with a heavy chair. Poor Harry was sitting on the toilet, lifeless. His head was bent forward on his chest, his corpulent body had prevented him from falling off the 'throne'.

I could not believe it. My head swam. I was losing patients at such a fast rate that if it continued at this pace I would have no practice left in three days! The two sisters who had followed me up the stairs did not appear to be as shaken as I was. I had indeed treated their two other brothers for heart trouble in the past, but never Harry! Harry had always been the well one.

They now seemed to take the whole ghastly happenings in their stride. Even the multi-symptomatic lady, who had spent her whole life moaning and groaning did not appear too upset. The youngest sister in the wheelchair when we came downstairs and told her the bad news simply looked at me and remarked, 'Can you arrange to have our brothers taken away before it gets dark?'

She apparently did not like to have dead bodies in the house after nightfall! Of the group who had survived the massacre in that house in Copleston Road that morning, I appeared to be the most upset.

While feeling sorry for the sisters who had lost three brothers on the same day, this sort of behaviour on the part of the doctor does not give one's practice a very good name. Patients are very reluctant to register with a doctor who appears to specialize in death, especially if he is in the wholesale business!

The coroner's officer to whom I reported the deaths listened to me in stony silence as I rattled off the names, one after the other. He retorted that it did seem a bit unusual to have three deaths in one house at the same time. I told him that I believed that they had all died of massive coronaries. I had already been treating two of the brothers for heart trouble for some time, and did not suspect anything unusual to be the cause of their deaths.

'What did they all have for breakfast?' he asked.

I had to admit I had not asked.

'Well, they could all have been poisoned, you know!'

I felt a fool! I hadn't thought about it.

He said that he would deal with the 'problem'. I could leave everything to him. He then rather punctiliously corrected himself; he would deal with the 'problems'. He would let me know the result of his findings in due course.

Post mortems were performed on all three brothers. I was wrong in one of my diagnoses. Only two of the brothers' deaths had been to be due to coronary thrombosis; the third had died as a result of a massive cerebro vascular accident.

The three sisters afterwards went on with their lives as though nothing untoward had happened. The multi-symptomatic sister continued to drive me mad with her various complaints, until she died in her eighties, of bronchopneumonia.

The fat sister suffered a stroke in her late seventies and departed this life in St Francis's Hospital, East Dulwich.

The youngest sister, the one who suffered from multiple sclerosis, I had to get admitted to a special home when her fat sister had a stroke; there was no one left at home to care for her.

13

Rogues' Solicitor

Mr Emmanuel Fryde, 'Manny', was an autocrat, and would never countenance any opposition to his dictat. He qualified as a solicitor in South Africa, but having matrimonial problems there, left to become domiciled in England. He never saw any reason to qualify in this country as he managed very well as the chief clerk of a law firm in the City. He ran the firm. He was the boss. Everyone knew it. The solicitors really worked for him, even though their names were on the letterheads.

Manny was flamboyant, an extrovert, domineering in his behaviour, miserly, but he could be benevolent whenever he felt like it. He was however superstitious to the point of stupidity and terrified of illness. He could have been called a hypochondriac, but this label did not quite fit his case for he never allowed his illnesses to interfere with his work schedule. He was a work-aholic.

My first encounter with him was in the South-East London Synagogue, New Cross, in 1956, when he was keen to be elected on to the board of management and canvassed for my vote. He was successful, became more and more outwardly religious, although his real aim was to become a warden of the synagogue. This he succeeded in doing at a later date.

His religious fervour knew no bounds, but it was selfish and irrational. It was a hypocritical farce, intensified as he grew older by his fear in the knowledge that he was approaching his day of judgment. Whilst pretending to be pious in the synagogue his bank manager spent Saturday morning placing bets on the races for him. This would even happen on Yom Kippur if there was a race meeting on.

He erected a *succah,* a booth for the Festival of Tabernacles, in the garden of his house in Pepys Road, but he did not use it. Although the festival lasts for seven days he spent this time in his flat in Brighton – with no *succah.* He knew before he had the *succah* erected that he intended to do this. He insisted that we knew about the *succah* however, by inviting me, my daughter, and the rabbi from Brighton to make a blessing in it, on a cold, dark, damp night. Manny came especially from his office for the five minutes we spent in it!

There is a special blessing to be made in a *succah* when one eats or drinks something in it, and Manny was not going to allow us to escape. It was pouring with rain; a *succah* having only a covering of leaves for a roof provided no shelter, and we were drenched to the skin. The rabbi who should have made the blessing seated, decided to forego this obligation, he would have had to sit in a pool of water. We left like drowned rats, and were rewarded for our 'piousness' with heavy colds!

One Saturday, at nine o'clock in the evening, in the winter of 1968, the telephone rang. It was Manny, with a request for me to go to West End Central Police Station to examine a client of his – immediately. The director of a large company had been charged for being drunk in charge of a car. There were no breathalyzers at that time and the standard tests were to speak to the accused, check for slurring of speech, and to ask the person to walk along a straight line.

When I arrived at the police station this client of his was sitting down in a cell. When I asked him to stand and walk along a straight line, he stood up, grabbed me around the waist, and began to waltz me around the room. The smell of his breath was so intoxicating that I had doubts whether I would be sober enough to drive home. I was only able to free myself with difficulty, and my struggles to do so only succeeded when he broke into hysterical fits of laughter. I just could not get any sense out of the chap. He was blind drunk, and I rang Manny to tell him.

He was disappointed. Couldn't I find any excuse for this unfortunate man's behaviour? He realized I had been disturbed on Saturday night and he was going to make sure that I was well-rewarded by his client for my visit.

My answer to him, 'My strictly orthodox upbringing will not allow me to lie in a situation like this,' appeared to please him. I was not asked to examine any of his drunken clients again although I knew he had many more cases of this type. He believed my behaviour was smoothing a path for him to heaven so he registered with me as a National Health patient! I rather stupidly accepted this heavy burden: I regretted it dozens of times but, to be honest, I was too afraid to refuse.

One lunchtime I was called to his firm to treat a racehorse trainer who was on a doping charge. It was an emergency, the patient was going to pay me privately, Manny had rung me himself to tell me so. Manny could never understand that there were other patients who demanded my attention more urgently. He never asked for a visit, he ordered one. The trainer had indeed collapsed in Manny's office, but on examination his symptoms proved to be an attack of nerves. Whether it was the fact that he was about to be charged by the police, or the fees that he was going to have to pay for legal advice, I did not stay to find out.

Even in 1970, it was difficult to park in the area of his office in St Bride's Street near Ludgate Circus, so when I stopped my car outside the door of his offices I was surprised to see a traffic warden waiting for me. I put my head out of the car window and asked him where to park.

'Right here,' he said.

He personally would watch after the car until I returned. He had been ordered by My Fryde's staff to watch out for me, to make sure that I did not receive a parking ticket.

Manny himself did not drive, but owned a chauffeur-driven car. Whether he had ever driven in this country I never found out and would never have had the audacity to ask him. His poor chauffeurs were bullied by him unmercifully, but the tips and pay made it worthwhile for a time until they could take his bullying no longer. They told me this themselves.

I was summoned at midnight one Saturday to witness Manny's signature to a document. This was an agreement between Manny and one of the popular Sunday newspapers to print the life story of Mr Wilson, one of the train robbers. Mrs Wilson had returned from Canada especially to give Manny written permission for the story to be printed. For these extra 'non doctoral' duties, at all times of the day or night, he carefully placed a five pound note in my top pocket before leaving.

A criminal at the top of his profession when apprehended by the police always asked for Mr Fryde to represent him. I remember seeing him on television going into Durham gaol to defuse a confrontation when the warders and prisoners did not see eye to eye. He was evidently regarded as the number one solicitor by the criminal fraternity, and apparently respected by the police!

The Kray brothers, some of the train robbers, and Nash, were amongst his 'clientèle'. I remember walking up the stairs in his house in Pepys Road late one night to attend his wife who was ill and being introduced to two men in evening dress who were coming down the stairs. Although he led an active social life he never allowed it to intrude on his work. These two young men were the Kray brothers, who made the headlines of the newspapers in the following week.

At his seventieth birthday party held at the King David Suite, Marble Arch, most of the tables were occupied by the chief detectives of Scotland Yard. He was on first name terms with them from the chief downwards. During the evening he proudly introduced me to a man whom he had that day successfully managed to get acquitted of a charge of murder. The man, accompanied by his wife, was in evening dress, and looked as if he wished he were a million miles away. They knew they were there just for Manny to show off.

As I have previously mentioned, he could at times be benevolent; this showed when he went to Israel on a group tour in 1970. He lost all reason! Like all Middle East countries, Israel at that time had its share of beggars, who seemed to have their own grapevine. They were out in force at every destination to greet him! The tour group travelled by bus, and when the bus reached one of the tourist sights and the occupants attempted to alight, the beggars were waiting. They pushed, jostled, and bruised every occupant who stood in their path to get to Manny. They appeared to recognize him, even knew him by name. The grapevine was faultless. He stood on the bus steps, and like an eastern potentate threw them five pound notes, like crumbs to birds. He was flamboyant, he thought that by this sort of charity he was buying himself a ticket to heaven.

His love of his fellow man and his fondness for me in particular was demonstrated when he telephoned me one morning about a year after his Israel trip to ask me to call and see him at his home on my way to the surgery. When I arrived at his home I found that I had been summoned to open a box of oranges, sent as a present to Manny by the speaker of the Knesset. Manny was giving me the honour of opening the box, on the lawn of his garden, and had prepared a hammer and screwdriver for the occasion. It was impossible for me to refuse to open the box and indeed, when opened, I found it contained top quality Jaffa oranges. I turned to give one to Manny, but he had disappeared; I finally found him cowering behind the settee in the lounge, some thirty feet from the box, and he showed not the least remorse as he proclaimed his friendship for me.

'Thank God! I thought the orange box might be booby-trapped and I didn't want to get blown to pieces!'

Manny was an enigmatic character, gave the appearance of being an observant and traditional Jew, but having divorced his first wife in South Africa, he married a long-suffering non-Jewish lady in this country. She was placid, docile, friendly and amiable: a character, in complete contrast to Manny. He dominated her completely, ruled every single action she ever undertook, and the only reward she received for her subservience was to live in luxury. She always took a back seat, she had no choice, but his behaviour gave her problems as he was also a womanizer. He once said to me when I dared to question his behaviour after he had contracted a urinary infection, 'My prick has no conscience.'

Mrs Fryde already had a daughter from her previous marriage, but this did not prevent him taking charge of the daughter's affairs, and of the daughter's children too. In fact he took total control of Mrs Fryde's family and gave them no opportunity to lead their own lives.

When Mrs Fryde's grandson married in Dulwich College Chapel Manny insisted that many of his own friends should be invited to the wedding, although they were unknown to the bride or groom. This must have been distressing to his wife's grandson and his bride as he had already interfered with their wedding plans. He had 'persuaded' the college chaplain to marry them on the day of his choosing, and they hated him for it. They were married in the chapel which was naturally their choice, after all, they were Christians, but were made to endure a reception and dinner held in the Café Royale under *kashrut* (rabbinical) supervision.

Mr Fryde, being the piper, called the tune!

Mrs Fryde often related to me of their experiences in eating out. Manny tried to give the impression of always eating *kosher,* and they regularly patronized Blooms in Whitechapel Road. He was already well-known there for his generous behaviour once he had drunk a few too many whiskies, and waiters waited expectantly for his arrival. When the Frydes arrived other diners would tend to be neglected for the waiters flocked around the Frydes like geese.

A waiter on seeing the Frydes arrive would immediately be despatched to the nearest off-licence to buy a bottle of whisky. They all knew that they would be well-rewarded for their attention to this detail. Poor Mrs Fryde then had the thankless task after his bout of heavy drinking of fending the waiters off, as they came back for their third, fourth, and fifth five pound tips.

His religious behaviour had some strange characteristics and his not being used to being contradicted led on one occasion to a very hostile reaction from a synagogue official. A fracas developed after a service, blows were struck over a trivial detail, and a lifelong enemy was made. He never forgot an insult, and spent his life making enemies. He carried to his grave enmity to people whom he thought had insulted him.

Another quirk to Manny's character was his fondness of birds. His budgerigar became indisposed, it refused to eat, so without hesitation a veterinary surgeon was called in. I visited Manny five days after the budgie had first taken ill and found the vet at Manny's home with the bird in his hand. He was dusting it down with a brush. He had been visiting daily to treat his patient and when I asked him what was wrong with the bird he said out of Manny's hearing, 'Nothing much.' The bird was moulting, but, 'If the bloke is a crank and wants me to come every day just to dust the bird down why should I turn good money away?'

His love of birds was quixotic. He would throw bread into his garden, then stand by his patio door anxiously waiting for them to come and eat. The first birds to arrive would always be wood-pigeons, just to annoy him. He would become hysterical, and run out screaming like a maniac to drive them away. He would become red in the face and speechless with rage. On the occasions I was present to witness these incidents I would have to calm him down, warning him of the effects these birds were having on his blood pressure.

One lovely, warm, August afternoon, I responded to a panic call to visit him at home. He was once again in a state of hysteria, and I found the house full of detectives and constables. Manny was running round the house like a man possessed. He had been on holiday, and on returning home had found to his horror that his home had been burgled. All Mrs Fryde's furs, including several minks had been stolen, but she was in no way as distressed as Manny. The thought that HE had been robbed by a criminal when he was the criminal's best friend was abhorrent to him. He just could not understand it. HE had actually suffered a burglary. Who could have done such a thing to him?

I learned some time afterwards that he had been burgled by a French gang who were not clients of his, not subject to his whims and pleasures. One sentence uttered by Manny on the telephone that day struck me very forcibly; I had no idea who he was talking to, but it sounded like one of his criminal fraternity.

'You don't have to go as far as that, you can let the bastards stay alive.'

Strange really, but it was the first and only time I ever heard him swear.

There was a clean-up in Scotland Yard in the 1970s and Manny decided it was healthier to leave the country posthaste. Before doing so however he went into hiding in this country, to give himself time to be able to remove files from his offices. Acting on a tip-off that his offices were about to be raided, he and an accomplice successfully removed vital evidence, which they subsequently burnt.

He fled to Majorca, and from there regularly phoned me at the surgery for medical advice on his symptoms: he said he did not trust the Spanish doctors. I believe he was just double-checking on the advice that he had been given. After having been diagnosed by me in one of these telephone consultations as having prostate trouble he decided to risk it, and come back to England to see a consultant of my choice.

He came over from Majorca at Easter time, on his own,

and was sheltered by Mrs Fryde's relatives. Easter that year coincided with Passover, and my children, who knew him well, will never forget his presence at our Passover *Seder* table.

He arrived at our house in Hillyfields Crescent, Brockley, on the first evening of Passover, dressed in a long overcoat, the collar of which was drawn up to his ears, a scarf over his mouth, and a trilby hat, the brim of which was pulled well down over his eyes. If ever there was a suspect, he looked like one in this outfit.

Before he left my house at midnight he dressed himself in this same fashion, turned to my children and said, 'They won't recognize me like this, will they?'

Who the 'they' were I have only recently found out. 'They' were the Regional Crime Squad and the Inland Revenue. After his Passover visit to England, having been diagnosed as being in need of a prostate operation, he returned to Majorca to settle some urgent business affairs before returning. He then came back to England to have the operation in the private wing of King's College Hospital.

I visited him in hospital on the first day after his operation, went to the private wing, but could not find him. By devious means, he had managed to get himself moved to a single room in the maternity block. He thought that if 'they' knew he was in England and in King's College Hospital they would not be able to find him. He must however have been the talk of every nurse in the hospital as his presence in that ward had certainly been known to the porter at the reception desk in the main building! He told me where Mr Fryde was without a second thought.

I went to the ward, but expressed no surprise at his accommodation. Knowing him as I did, the last thing I would have said to him is, 'Where is the baby?'

After his operation he went back to Majorca. After some years he decided that the 'climate' in this country had changed enough for his safe return. He came back to live, and die, in Brighton. Thank heavens he was too old to visit me, and my practice was also too far for me to agree to be his doctor.